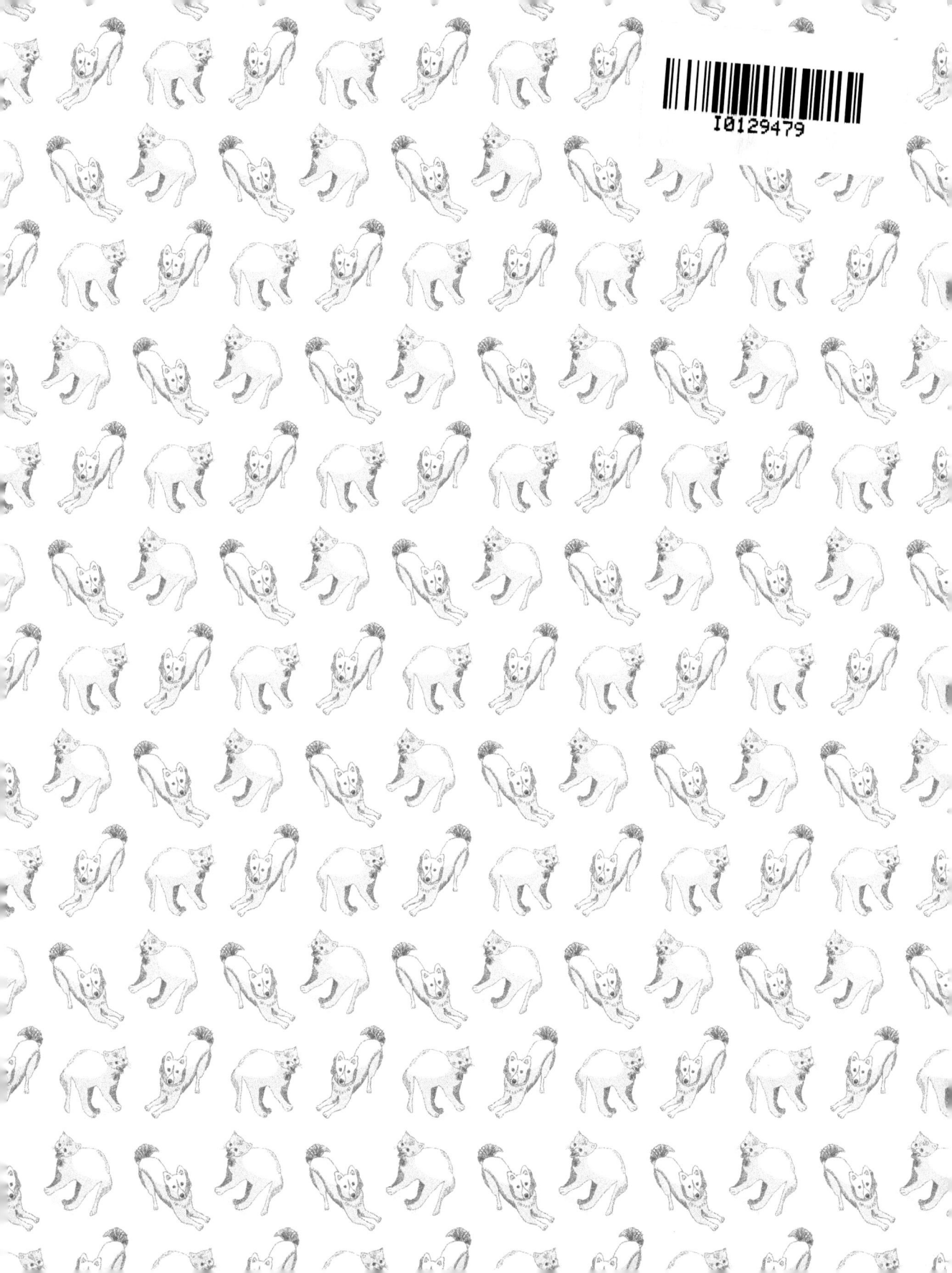

Cats as well as other animals acquire this ideal rhythm of motion because they are constantly stretching and relaxing themselves, sharpening their claws, twisting, squirming, turning, climbing, wrestling, and fighting.

Also observe, too, how cats sleep – utterly relaxed whether they happen to be lying on their back, side or belly. Contrology (Pilates) exercises emphasize the need for this constant stretching and relaxing.

Joe Pilates in *Return to Life Through Contrology*

THE PILATES ANIMALS WORKOUT

Exercise That Helps You Feel as Fit as an Animal

THE PILATES ANIMALS WORKOUT

Exercise That Helps You Feel as Fit as an Animal

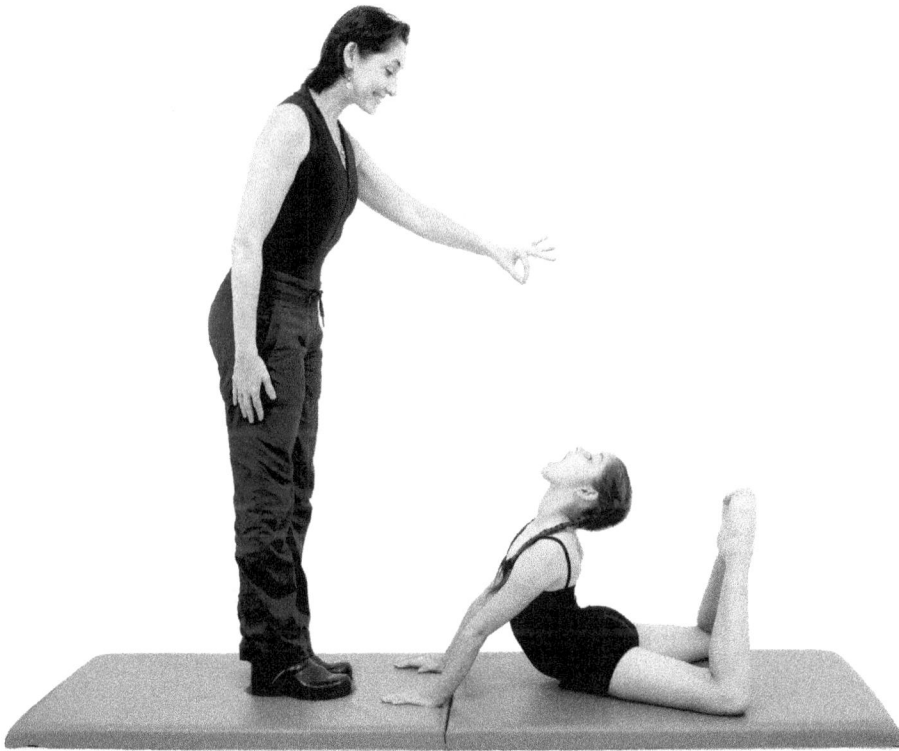

Written by Christina Maria Gadar
Illustrated by Taís Haydée Gadar

Gadar, Christina Maria.
The pilates animals workout: exercise that helps you feel as fit as an animal. /
Christina Maria Gadar
ISBN: 978-1-7337864-2-3

Illustrations: Taís Haydée Gadar
Photography: Max Kelly
Interior Book Design: Yael Rotstein Campbell
Cover Design: Max Kelly
Models: Marcelo Gadar, Taís Haydée Gadar, Christina Maria Gadar
Pilates Mat: Gratz Industries

To order more copies of *The Pilates Animals Workout*, visit:
www.PilatesPersonalTraining.com

Dedication

For all the pets that made my childhood extra special,

For my angels Paquita, Xuxa, and Marshmallow,

For my four legged family members
Pirlimpimpim,
Leila Rose,
Toby Royal Blue,
J.J. "Pipoca" Awesome
Penelope Sunshine,
Odin Filippovich,
and Vili Manili.

For all the animals who are yet to enter my life,

And for all the humans who adopt and foster animals from rescue organizations.

> *When I was eight years old I didn't play like other children. My fun was in watching people and studying them. I began studying animals, too, those in the zoo as well as those in the wilderness. I soon discovered that animals had a wonderful system of keeping fit. You never see a big cat out of shape. With just a little daily stretching and balancing on the rocks and benches in its cage, a lion or a tiger keeps itself in condition.*

Joe Pilates in an interview with *Pageant*

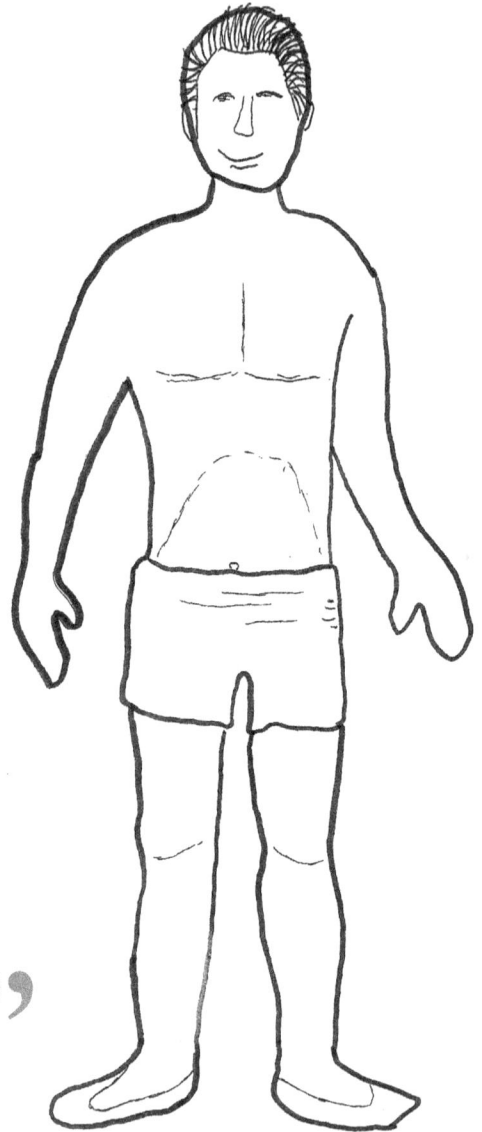

Who Was Joe Pilates?

Joe Pilates (pi-LAH-teez) was born in Germany and studied the movement of wild animals in nearby forests from the age of eight. His fascination with animal movement helped him move naturally and improved his ability to perform the gymnastic moves his father taught him. Later, he became a circus performer.

While in England during World War I, Joe was put in an internment camp. At the internment camp, Joe noticed that the stray cats were dealing with the lack of nutrition and less than ideal living conditions better than many of the people. With not much else to do, Joe observed the cats for hours on end and came to the conclusion that their constant stretching was a key factor in their ability to adapt to their surroundings.

Joe decided that he could help the other prisoners stay strong physically and mentally by teaching them exercises inspired by his observation of animals and his gymnastics training. Not one of his fellow prisoners died from the influenza pandemic in 1918 that spread a deadly flu virus across the world. During the four and a half years he spent in the internment camp, Joe began to develop a system of physical and mental conditioning that would change the lives of many people for years to come.

After the war, Joe returned to Germany. When he was in his early 40's, he moved to New York and began teaching the public his system of exercises designed to correct posture and energize the body. One of his biggest dreams was to have his Method incorporated into the education system for children.

How to Use This Book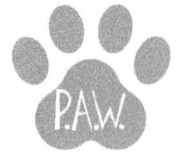

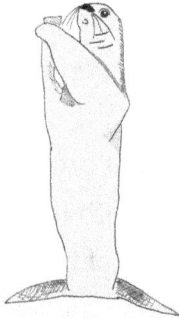

1 The Pilates Animals Workout® presents Joe's original work in a creative way that captures the imagination of children and leaves them feeling as fit as animals. It was created for children, but it can be done by anyone who wants to move like an animal!

Before teaching your children movements from the Pilates Animals Workout®, please take time to read the exercise descriptions, study the corresponding photos, and try the movements yourself. **2**

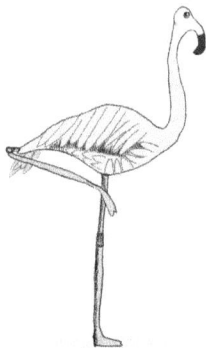

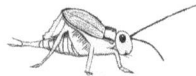

3 You can guide children through the animal movements or perform the exercises with them.

The Pilates Animals Workout® can be done in the order presented here. But if you would like to change the order, that's okay, too.

4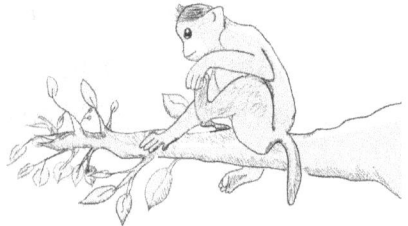

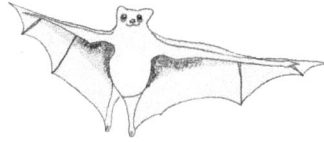

5 The Pilates Animals Workout® can be done in its entirety, or you can focus on a small group of exercises.

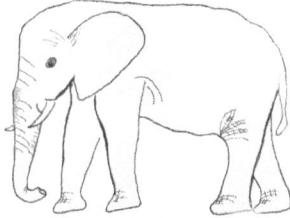

Each P.A.W. exercise is introduced with an illustration of the animal that inspired the movement and an interesting animal fact, followed by two exercise descriptions and accompanying photos. Based on what is most suitable for you and/or your child, pick either the introductory sequence or the more challenging sequence. **6**

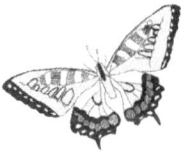

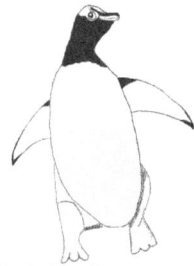

7 If an exercise doesn't feel right for your body or seem right for your child, skip it and move on to the next exercise. A good rule of thumb is to leave it out if you have a doubt.

Use your imagination as you do the Pilates Animals Workout® and you'll discover that it's fun to be as fit as an animal! **8**

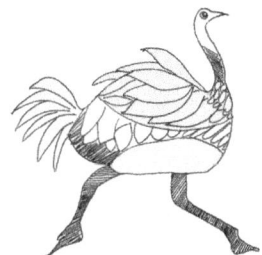

Introducing
The Pilates Animals Workout®

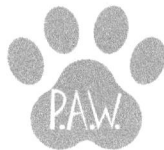

The Animals

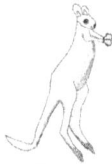

1

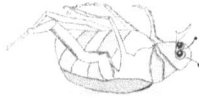

2

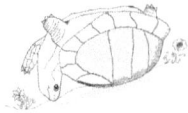

3

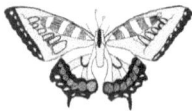

4

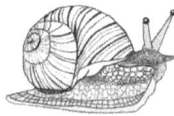

5

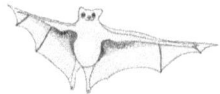

6

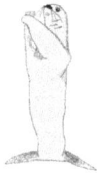

7

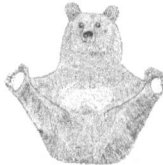

8

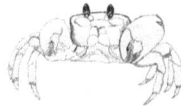

9

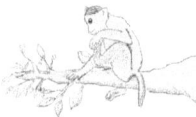

10

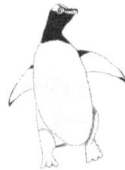

11

12

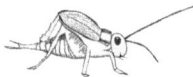

13

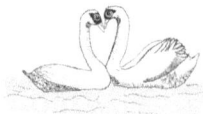

14

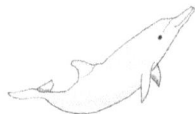

15

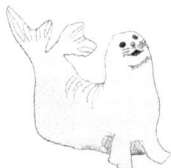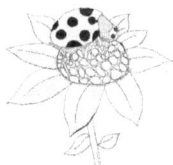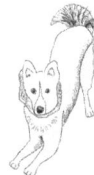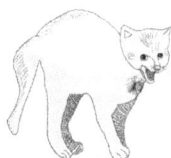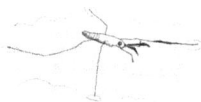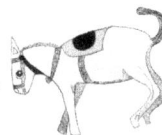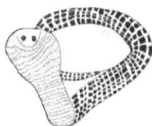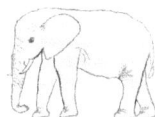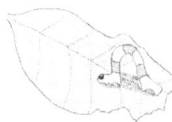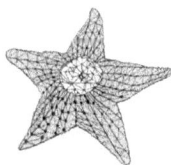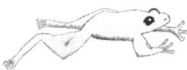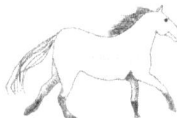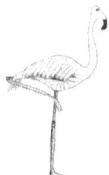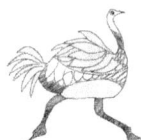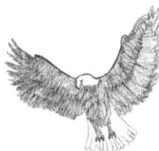

The Movements

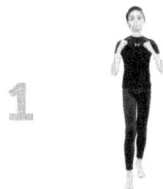

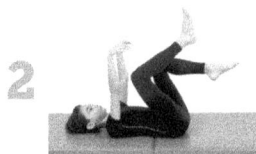

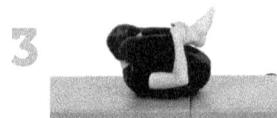

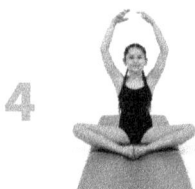

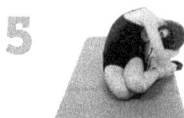

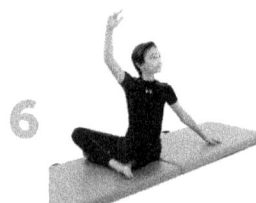

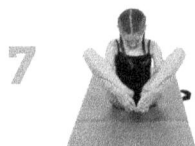

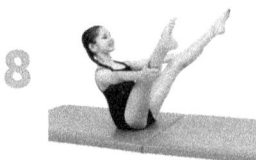

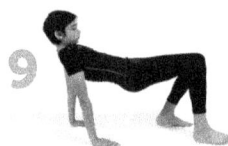

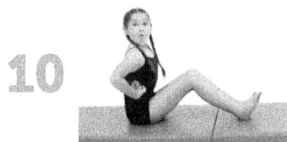

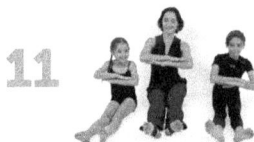

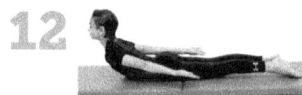

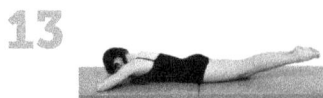

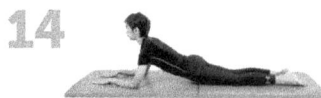

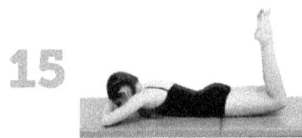

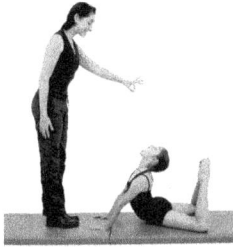

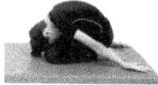

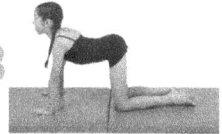

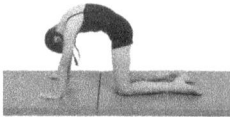

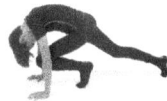

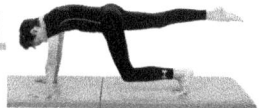

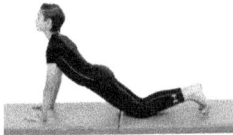

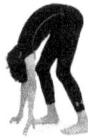

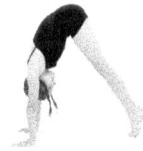

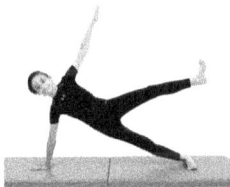

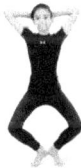

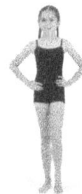

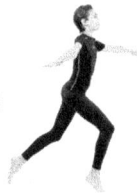

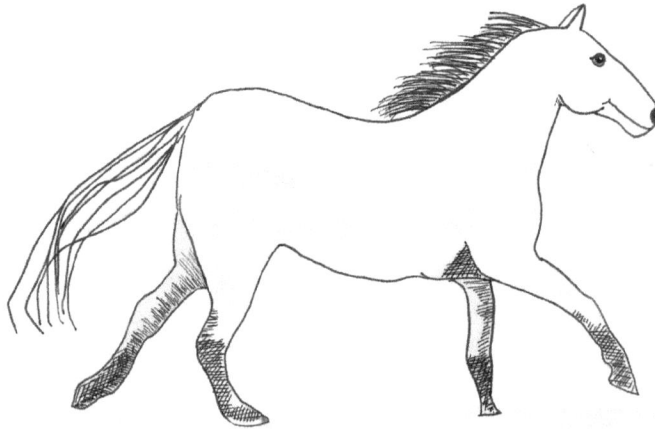

Take a horse, if a man wants to race him, he keeps him in top form. He makes the horse move. Why not keep humans in top form, too?

Joe Pilates in an interview with *The New York Times*

The Pilates Animals Workout®

Animal Facts and Movement Descriptions

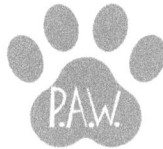

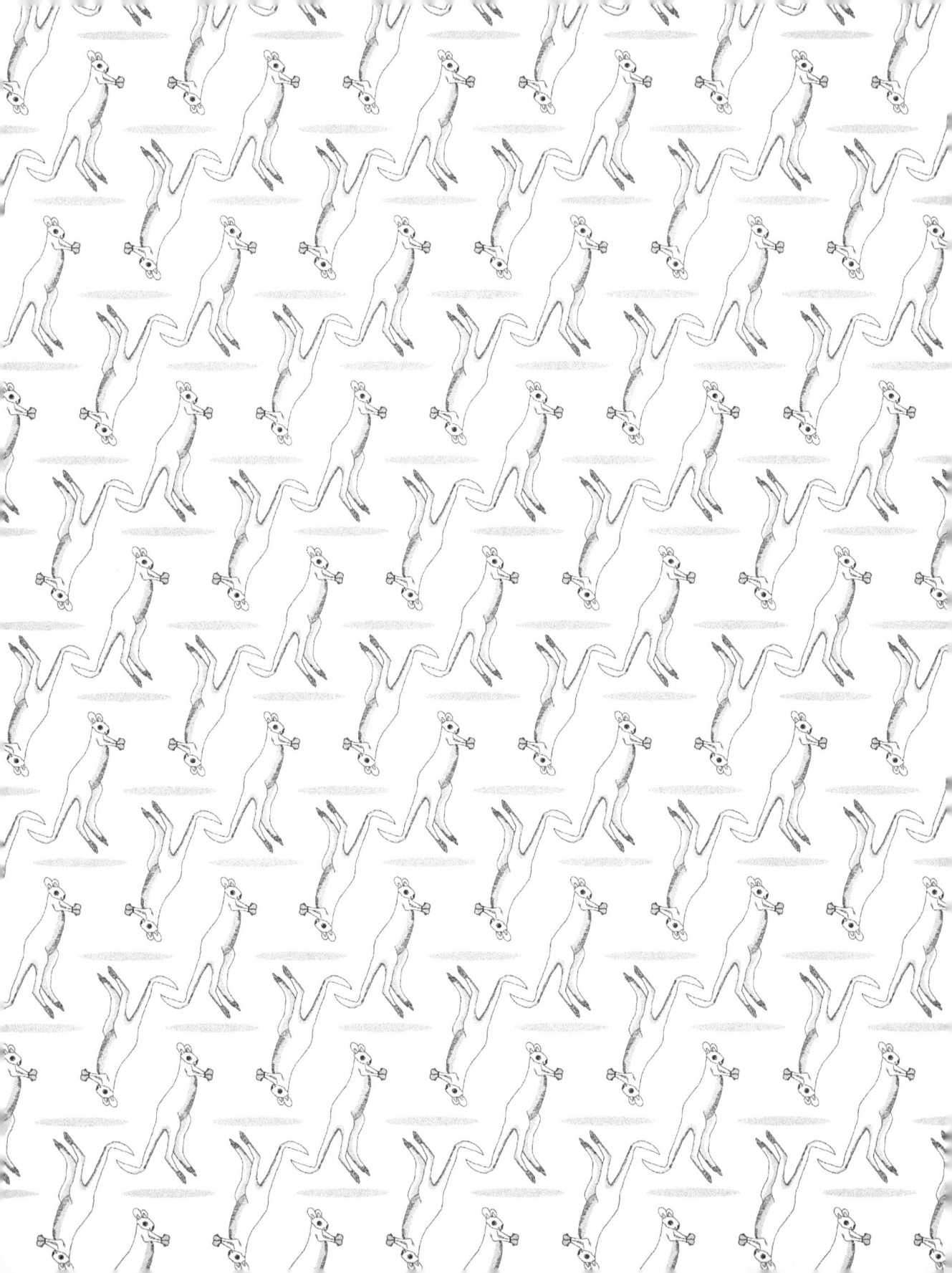

Kangaroo

Male kangaroos "box" each other with their forelegs, which resemble arms, to establish dominance. They can also balance all their weight on their tails as they kick their hind legs at the same time.

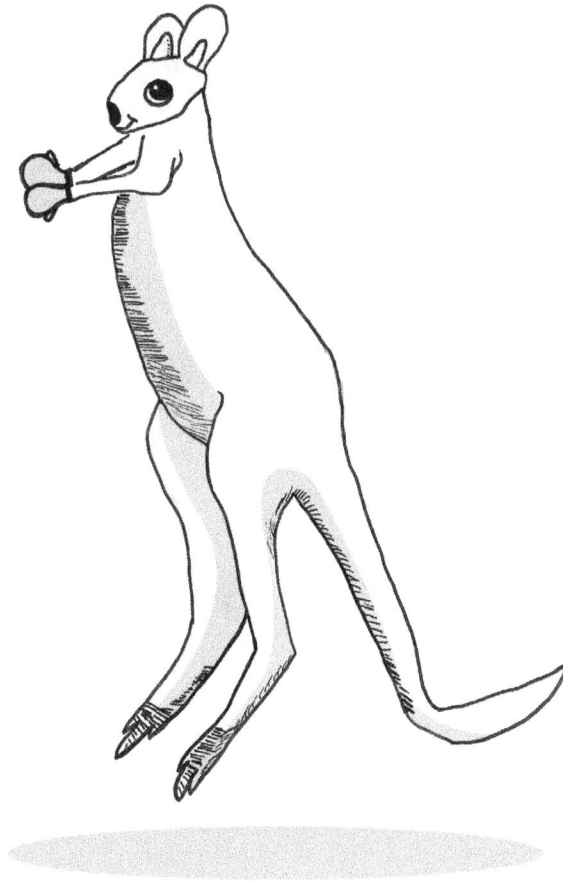

Boxing Kangaroo

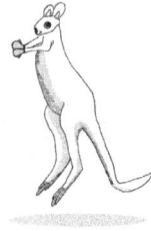

Starting Out

- Stand with your feet together, and your stomach muscles pulled in and up as if you are zipping up tight pants.

- With your hands curled into fists, bend your arms and tuck your elbows into your sides, slightly behind your waist. *Pretend you are a kangaroo preparing to throw a punch.*

- Alternate jumping your legs out and in, as in jumping jacks. **Photo A**

- Perform 20 times.

A

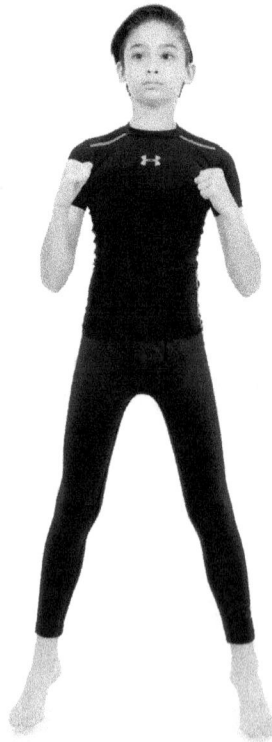

Deeper Practice

- Jump your feet out and in, as in a jumping jack movement 10 times. **Photo A**

- Then do small jumps with one leg in front and one leg behind. After 6 jumps, repeat with the other leg in front for 6 more times. **Photo B**

- Then jump 8 times alternating legs front and back.

- Then jump with the feet together 8 times.

B

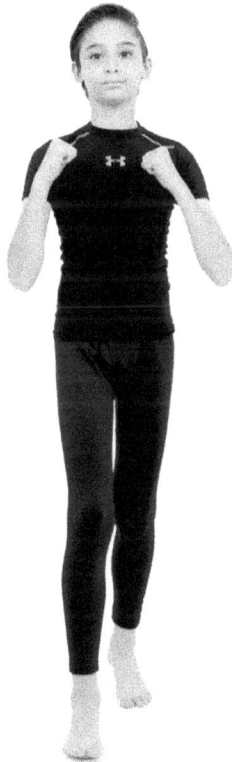

Bug

A bug carries the majority of his body weight near the top of his rounded body and must continuously use his little leg muscles to stay upright. Essentially, a bug is constantly doing push-ups to keep from tipping over!

Rest your arm on a table with your palm facing up. Notice how your fingers curl when your hand is relaxed. When a bug goes into a relaxed state, his limbs will also curl, causing him to topple over onto his back.

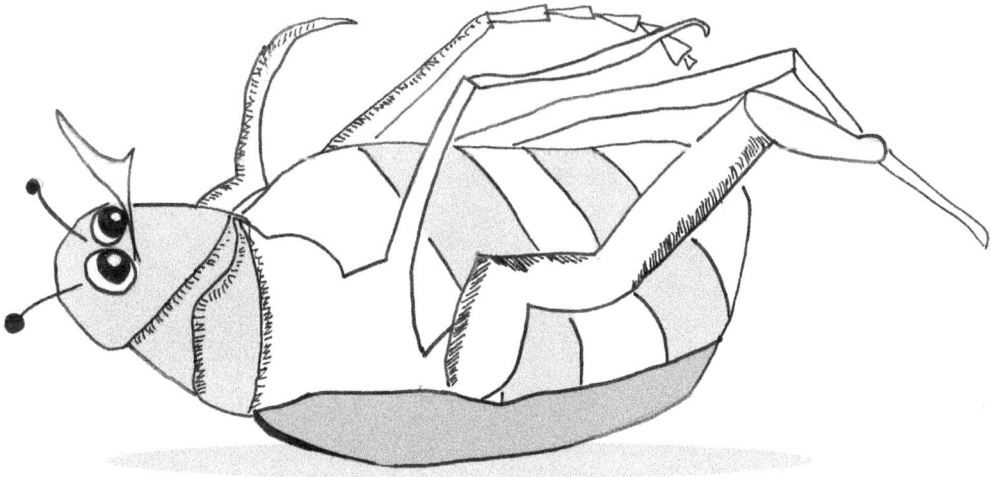

Dead Bug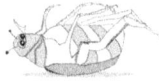

Starting Out

- Lie on your back and extend your limbs toward the ceiling.

- Gently shake them out. **Photo A**

- *Imagine you are a bug who has tipped over because you can no longer tense your leg muscles.*

A

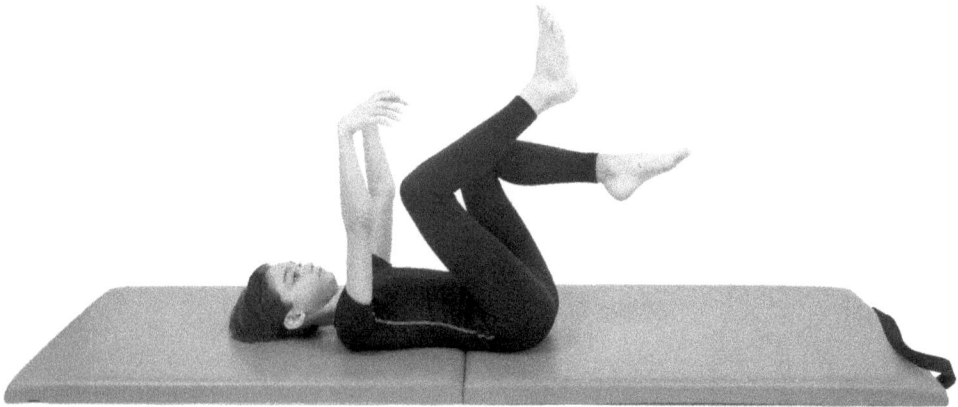

Deeper Practice

- Lie on your back with your legs bent at a ninety-degree angle, feet in the air.

- Lift your head and look at your bellybutton.

- Extend your arms long by your sides and pump them up and down.

- Breathe in for the first five pumps and breathe out for the next five pumps. **Photo B**

- Pump your arms up to 100 times as you breathe in and out.

B

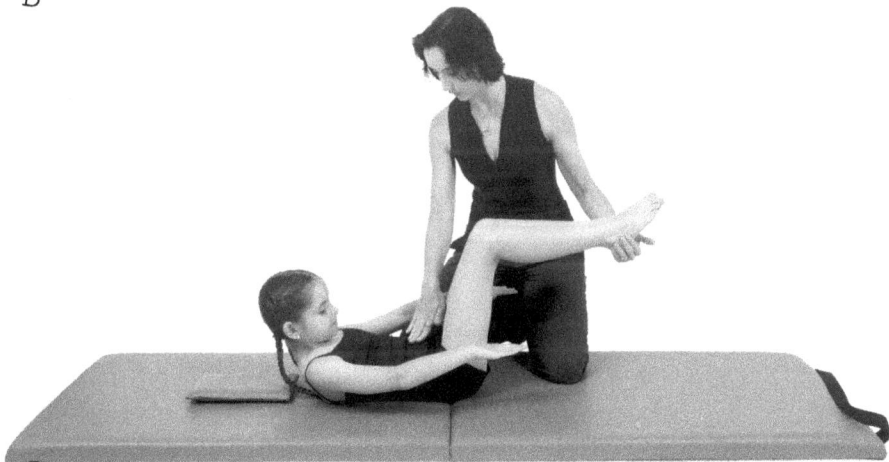

Turtle

Land turtles have much shorter legs and necks than sea turtles, making it harder for them to flip over after getting stuck on their backs. A turtle stuck on its back could die from starvation or exposure to the sun, so it is important to have an adult turn the turtle right side up.

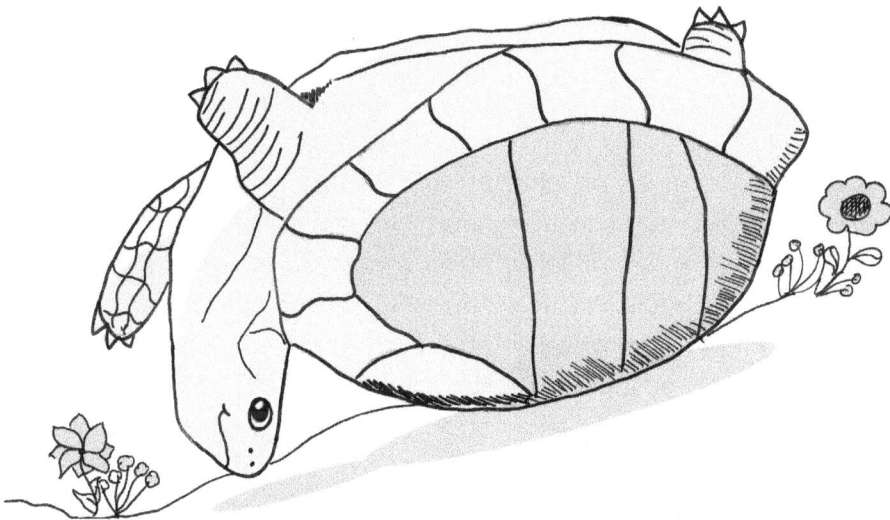

Turtle on its Back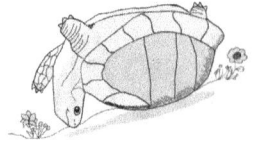

Starting Out

- Lie on your back and bend your knees into your chest.

- Pull your bellybutton into the mat and lift your head as you look toward your bellybutton.

- Hold the backs of your thighs or the front of your ankles.

- Try to bring your nose between your knees, while keeping your heels together and your knees slightly apart. **Photo A**

- Hold the ball shape for the count of "one Pilates, two Pilates, three Pilates," before resting the back of your head on the mat.

- Perform up to 3 times.

A

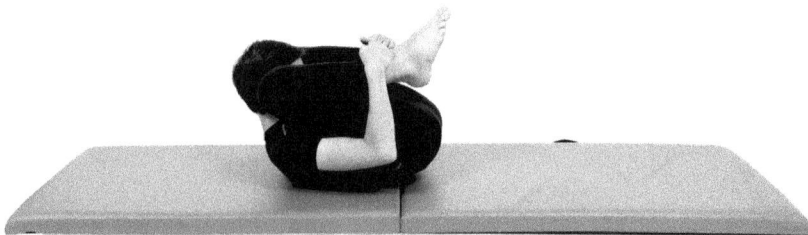

Deeper Practice

- Sit on the mat and make a ball shape by drawing your knees to your chest, feet to your seat, and your head between your knees.

- Hold the backs of your thighs or the front of your ankles.

- Try to balance with your feet above the mat. **Photo B**

- In time, you can attempt to roll like a ball, with even pressure on both sides of your spine.

- Be sure not to let the back of your head touch the mat as you roll back.

- After you roll onto your back, make three honest attempts to roll up again while holding your ball shape. **Photo C**

- *You might feel like a turtle struggling to flip upright after getting stuck on your back, but it is okay if you do not make it all the way up to the seated position.*

B

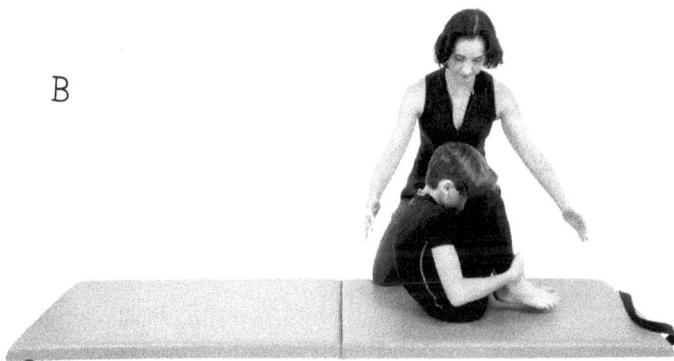

C

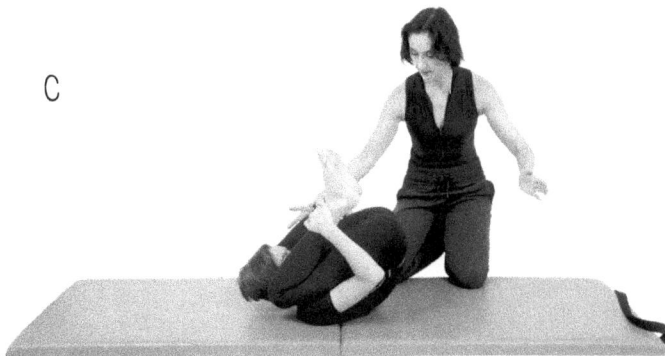

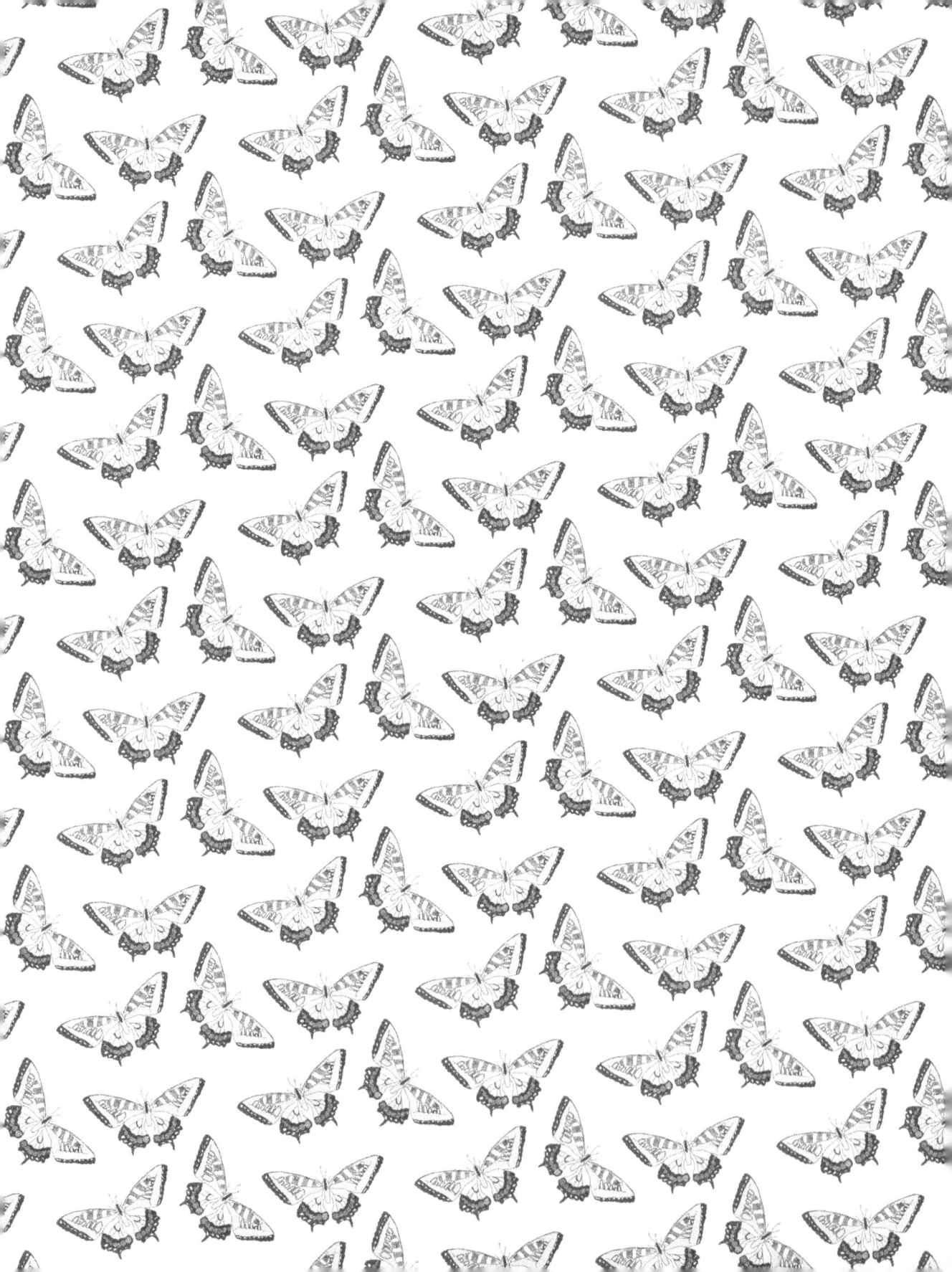

Buttferfly

A swallowtail butterfly uses the sensory hairs on her feet to taste up to six different substances. As she walks on leaves, a swallowtail butterfly can even determine the age and health of a plant. Knowing these things helps her decide where to lay her eggs so that her freshly hatched caterpillars will have immediate access to tasty, juicy leaves.

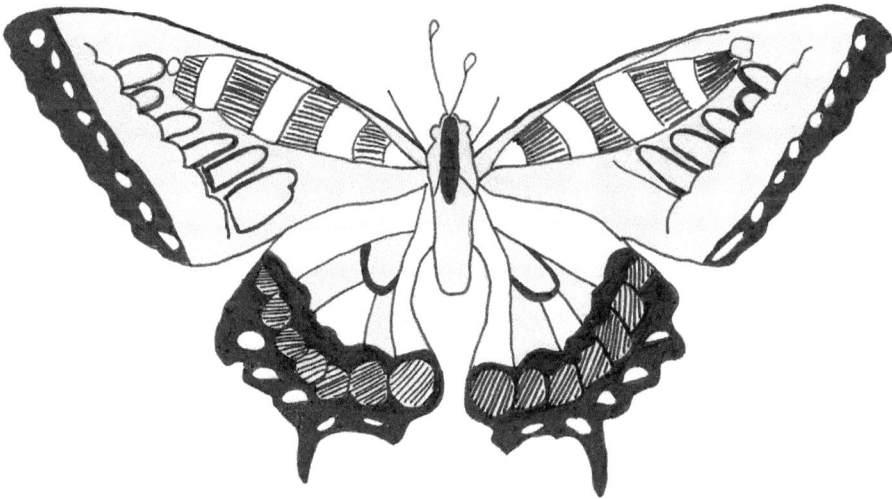

Buttferfly Wings

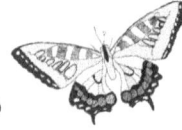

Starting Out

- Sit tall and bend your legs so that the soles of your feet come together and your knees open. **Photo A**

- *To mimic the flutter of butterfly wings in flight, hold your ankles and gently move your knees up and down.*

A

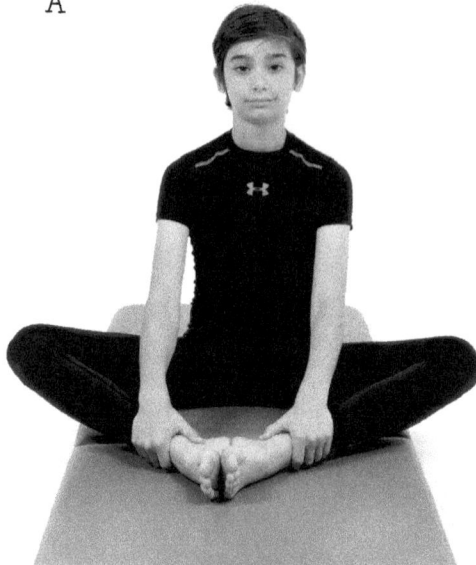

Deeper Practice

- Sitting with legs bent in the butterfly position, extend your arms forward as you bend at the waist. **Photo B**

- As you roll up from your forward bend, lift your arms so that they frame your face. **Photo C**

- To complete the arm circle, place your hands on the floor slightly behind you and lift your chest up toward the ceiling. **Photo D**

- Perform 3 times.

B

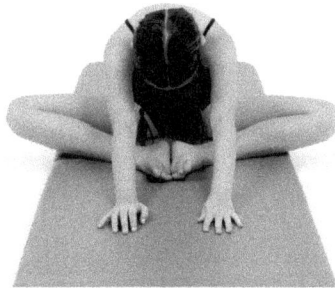

C

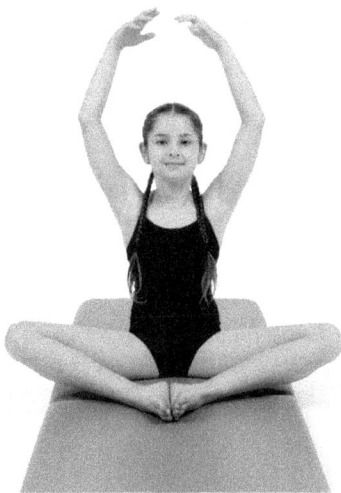

D

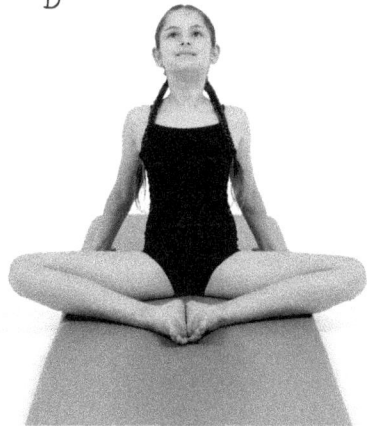

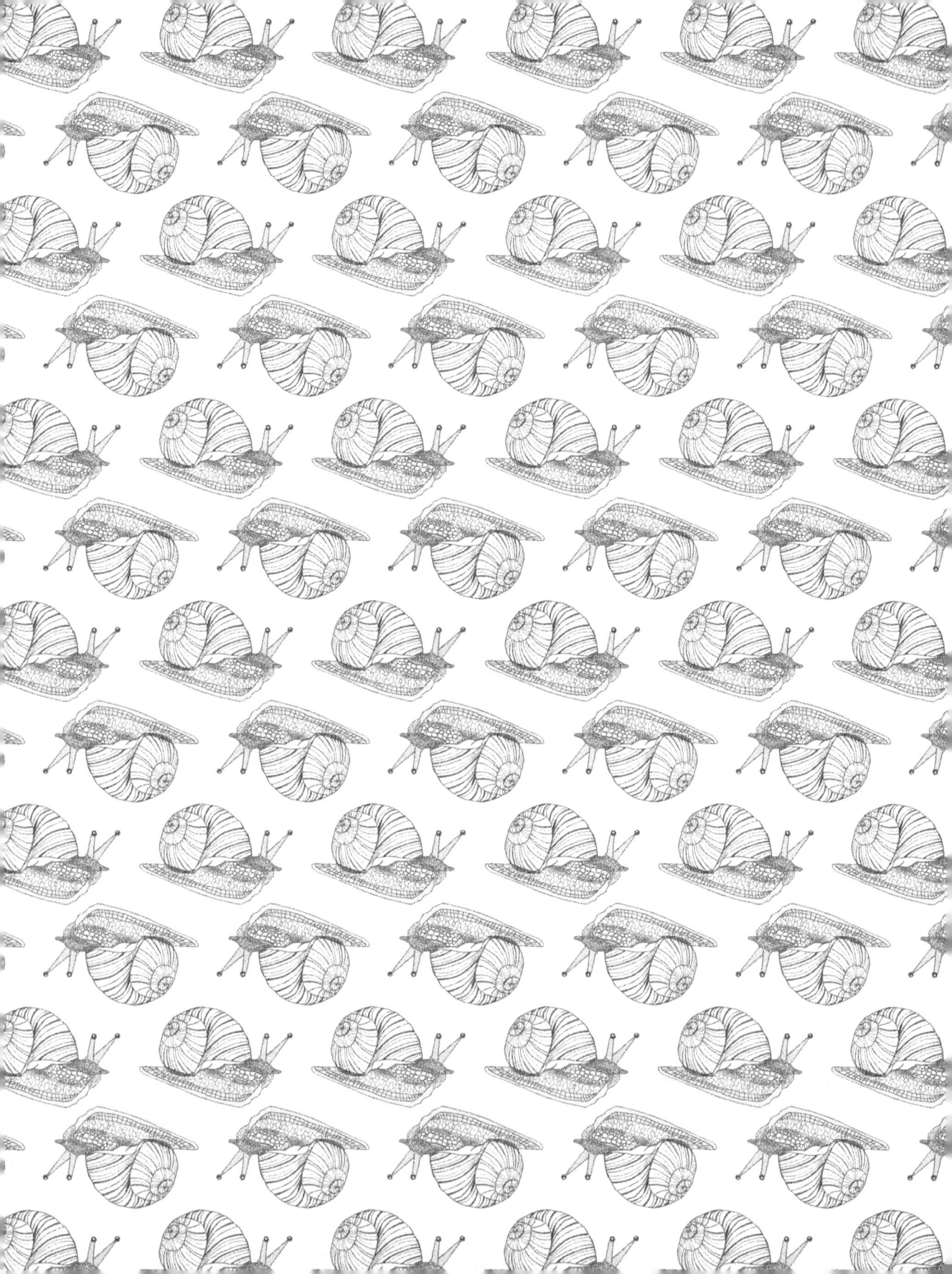

Snail

A baby snail usually begins its calcium-rich diet by eating the shell of the egg it hatched from. As the snail continues to grow, its own shell grows with it.

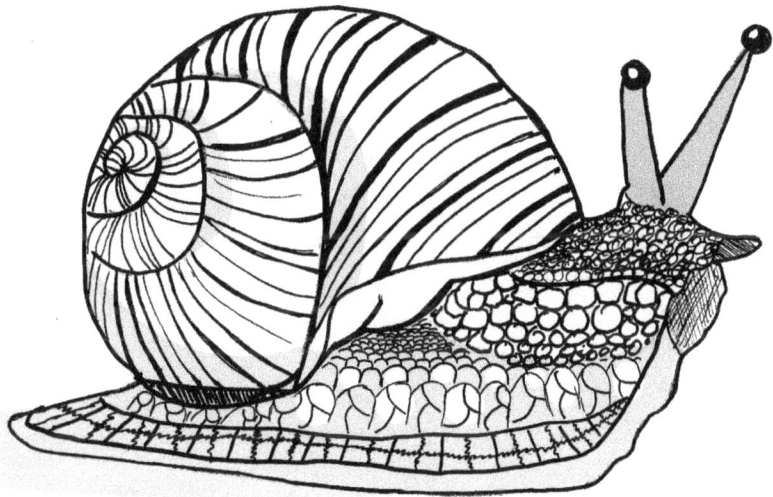

Snail Shell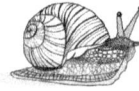

Starting Out

- Sit tall and take the "criss-cross applesauce" position, with your legs bent and crossed.

- Hold the front of one ankle with one hand and extend the other arm upward.

- Bend your body to the side, away from your raised arm. **Photo A**

- To deepen the side stretch, fold your top arm around your head. **Photo B**

- To work the waist, twist your body, bringing your top elbow toward your opposite knee. **Photo C**

- *Imagine that you are curling into a tiny snail shell as you twist from your waist.*

- To come out of the stretch, twist back to face the front of the room. Stretch your top arm and sit tall.

- Repeat on the other side.

A

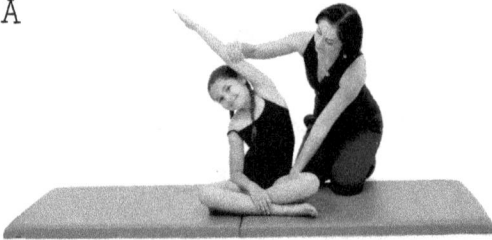

B

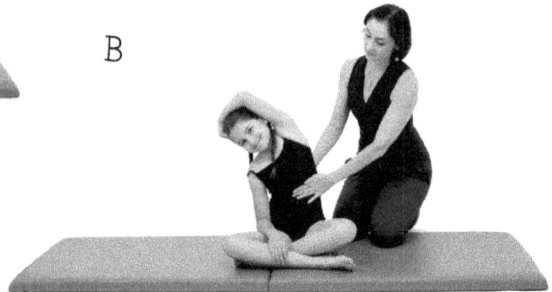

C

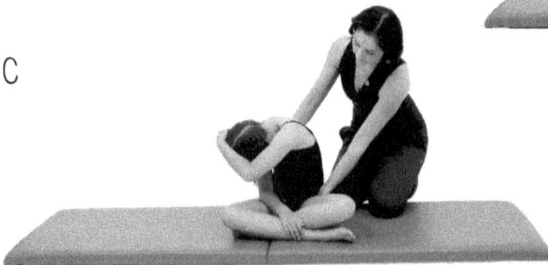

Deeper Practice

- Try the same exercise while sitting on one hip with your legs bent and stacked to the other side of your body.
- The hand closest to the feet holds the top ankle and the other arm extends upward. **Photo D**
- Bend your body toward your legs, and fold your top arm around your head. **Photo E**
- Twist toward your legs and bring your top elbow toward your knees. **Photo F**
- Twist back toward the front, stretch your top arm and sit tall.
- Repeat with the legs stacked on the other side of the body.

D

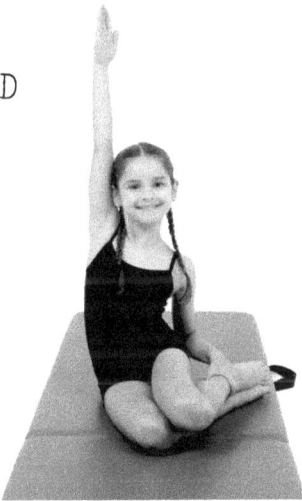

E

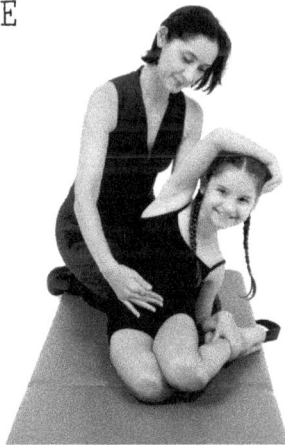

F

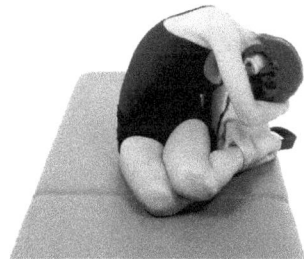

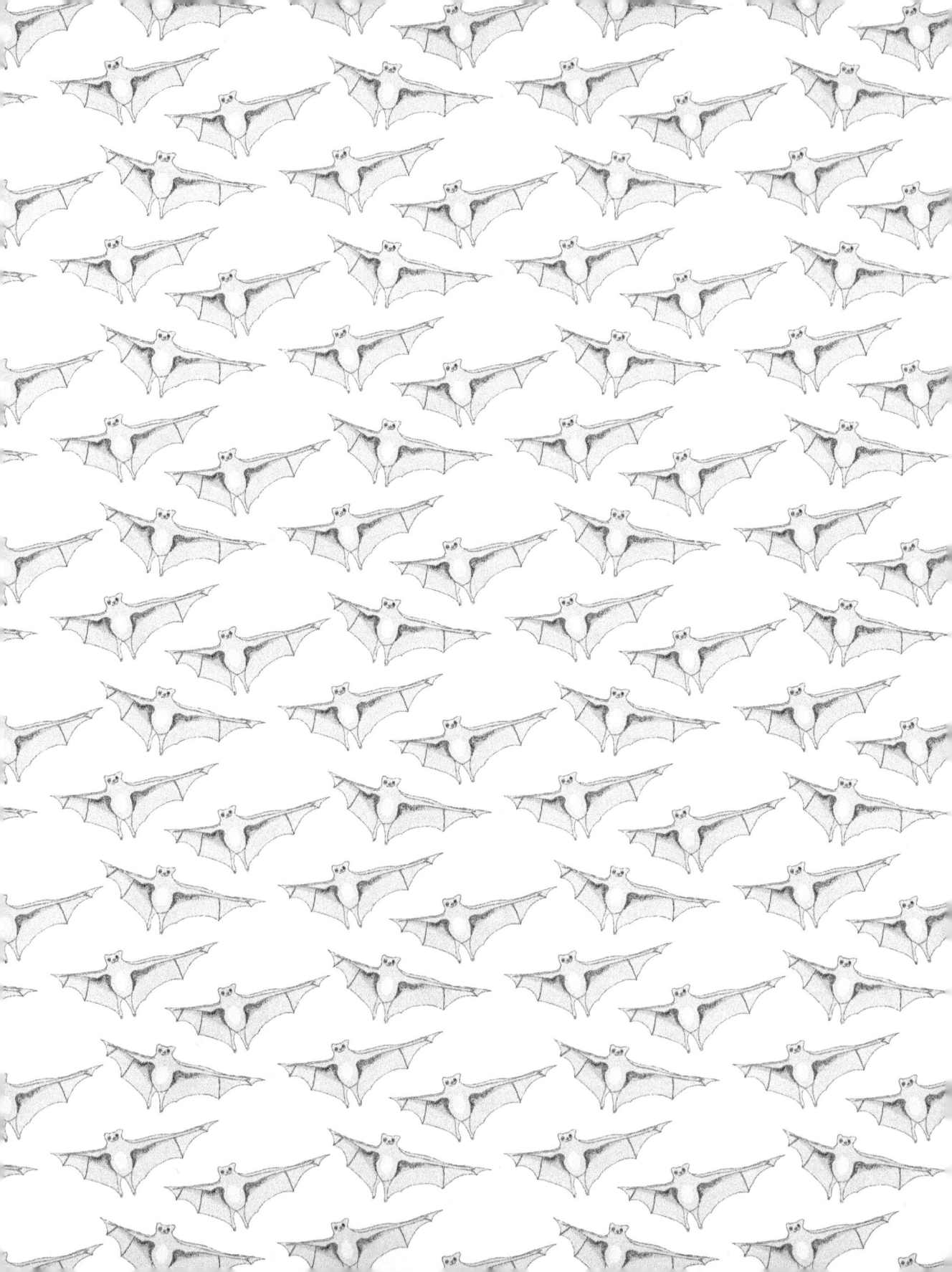

Bat

Unlike birds, the wings of bats are not designed for take off, and their feet (talons) are not designed for perching. To initiate flight, bats have to launch themselves from a high location. This might be the reason why bats sleep upside down. If they are hanging from their feet, all they need to do is let go, spread their wings, and they are instantly flying.

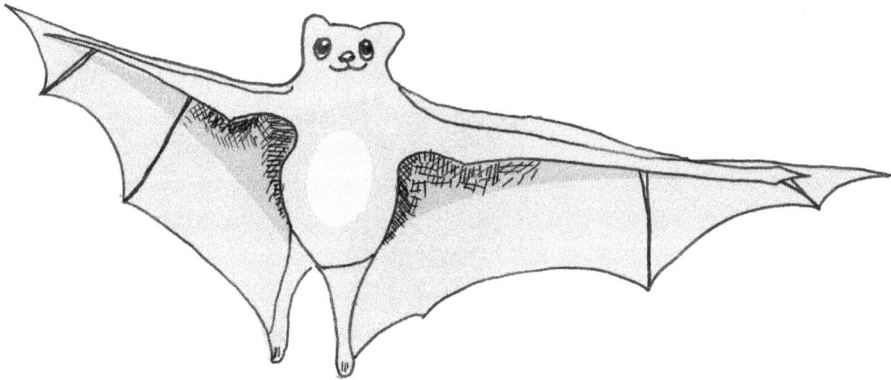

Bat Wings

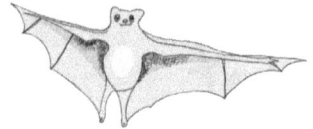

Starting Out

- Sit in "criss-cross applesauce" position, with your legs bent and crossed.

- Extend your arms out to the sides of the room and take a deep breath. *Imagine you are a bat, spreading your wings to take flight.*

- As you twist tall from your waist, let your breath out. **Photo A**

- Do 1 twist on each side and repeat another set with the other leg crossed in front.

A

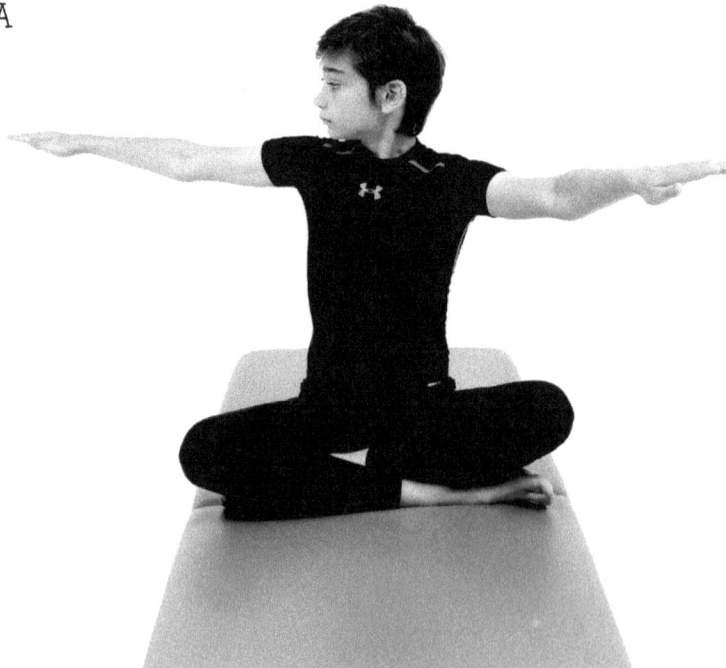

Deeper Practice

- Sit in "criss-cross applesauce" position with your legs bent and crossed.

- Extend your arms out to the sides of the room and take a deep breath.

- Twist from your waist as you breathe out.

- While still breathing out, look over your shoulder and put the palm of the back hand behind you on the floor, keeping your arm straight as the front arm reaches upward, next to your face. **Photo B**

- Do 1 twist on each side and repeat another set with the other leg crossed in front.

B

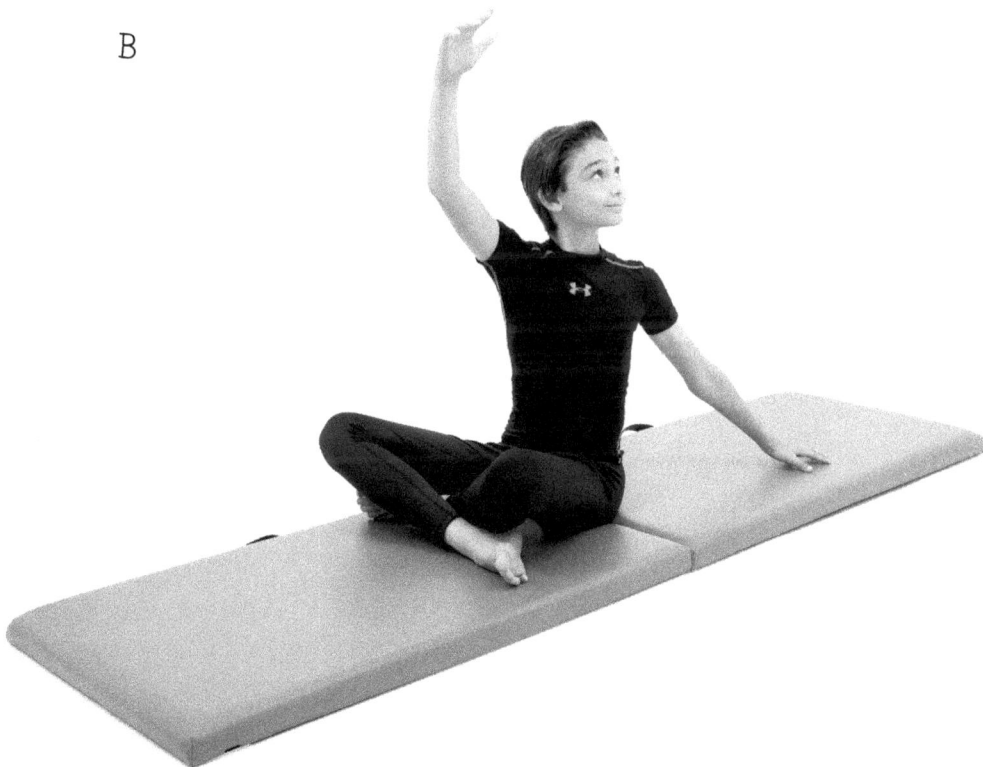

Sea Lion

You might think of seals when you think of those marine mammals at the aquarium that are trained to clap their flippers, but those are actually sea lions. Although both seals and sea lions can move in and out of the water, sea lions have large flippers that can be used for walking on land while seals have very small flippers that make them better adapted to the water. Sea lions are extremely intelligent and those held in captivity can be trained to do many tricks.

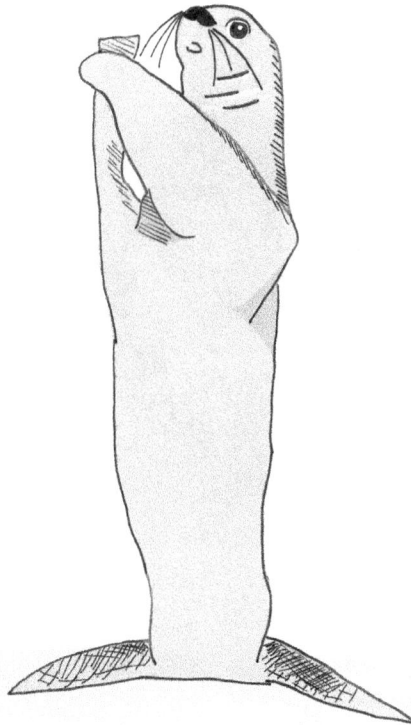

Playful Sea Lion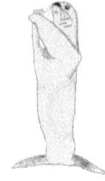

Starting Out

- Sit with the inner edges of your feet touching each other and hold your ankles, with your thumbs on the inside and your fingers on the outside.

- With your knees on the outside of your arms, shift your center of gravity back and balance with your toes slightly above the floor. **Photo A**

- *Imagine that your feet are flippers as you use your inner thighs to clap the inner edges of your feet three times.*

- Rest the feet and repeat 2 more times.

A

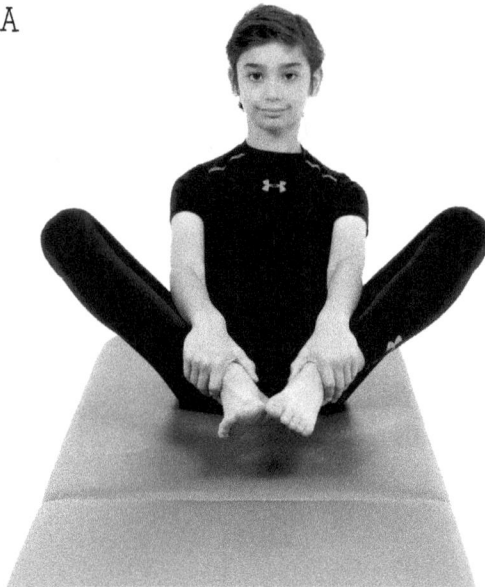

Deeper Practice

- Sit with the inner edges of your feet touching each other and put your elbows between your legs.

- Wrap your hands around the backs of your ankles, resting the palms of your hands on the tops of your feet with your fingertips pointing toward your toes.

- After finding your balance with your toes off the floor, clap the inner edges of your feet three times. **Photo B**

- Rest the feet on the floor, then repeat 2 more times.

B

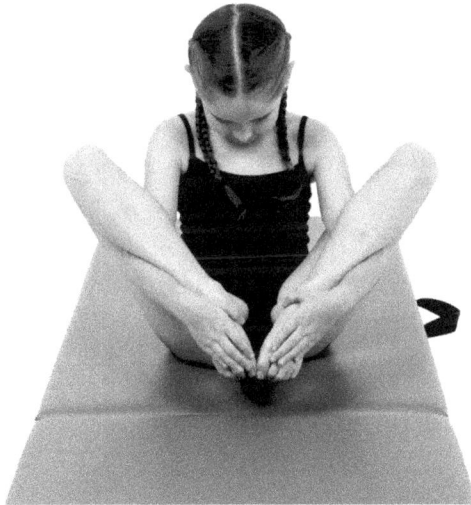

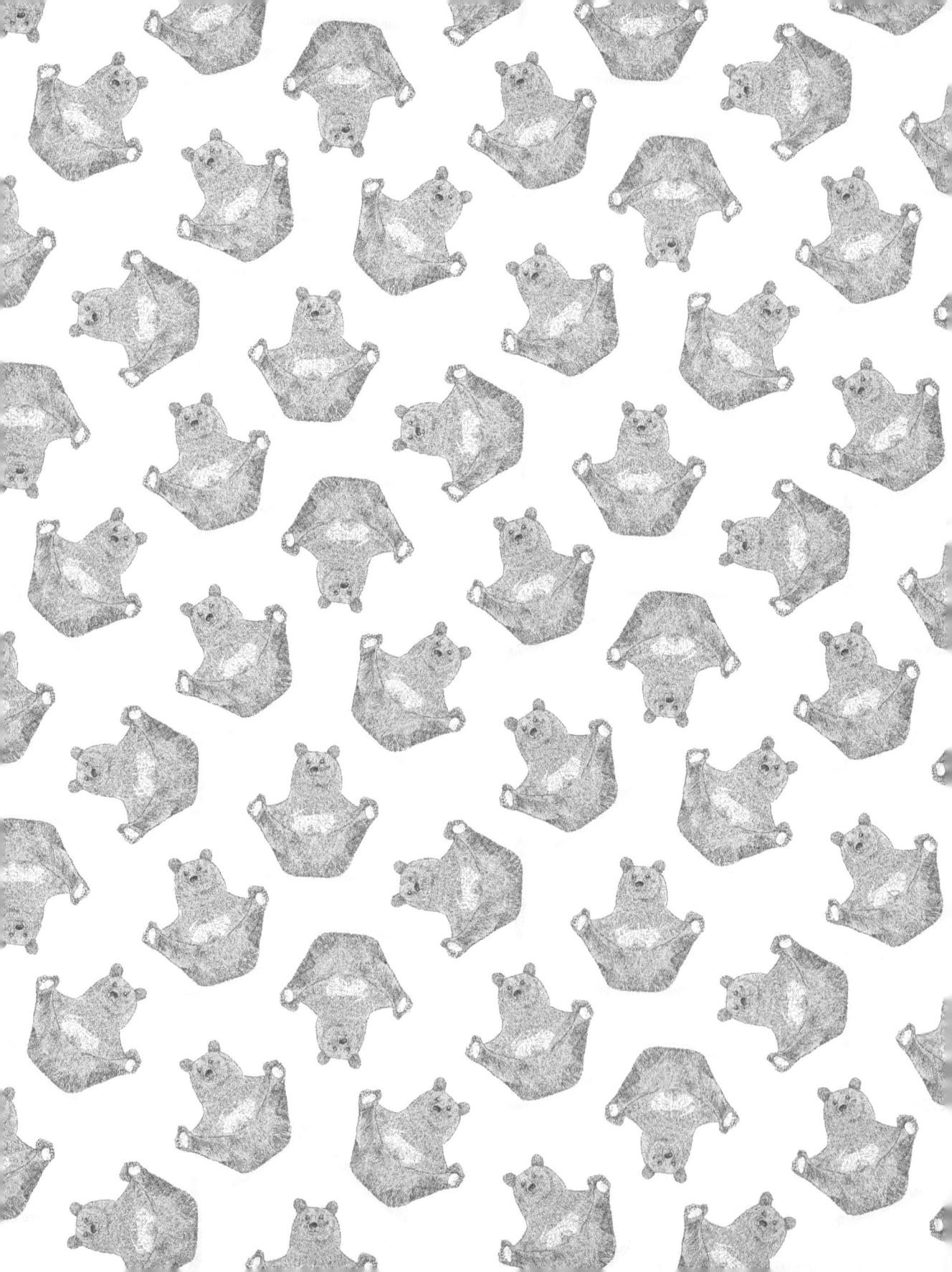

Bear

The melting of the Arctic sea ice is causing grizzly bears and polar bears to come into contact with one another. Grizzly bears previously identified as blond grizzlies are now being identified as the offspring of polar bears and grizzly bears, known as pizzly bears.

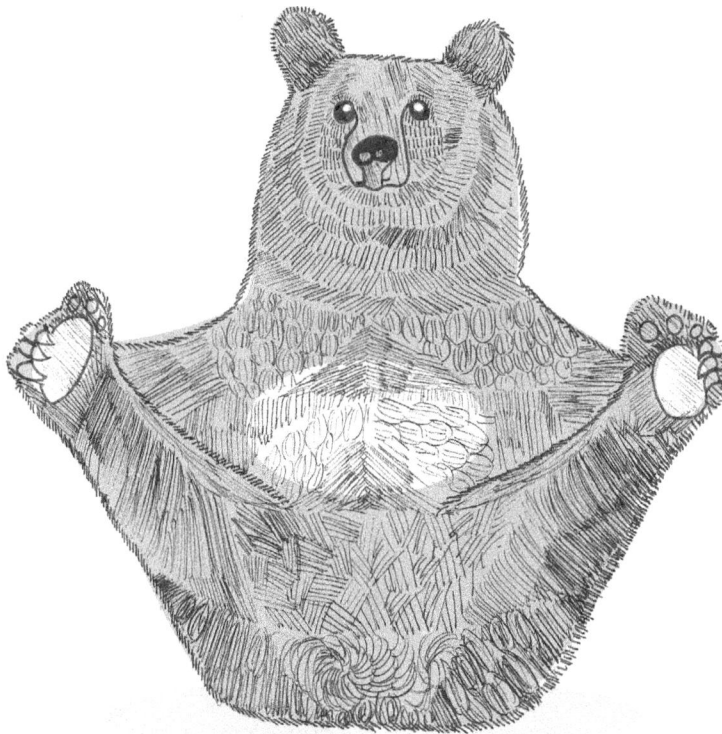

Grizzly Bear

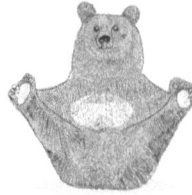

Starting Out

- Sit with bent legs, knees apart, and the toes of both feet touching each other on the mat.

- Pull your bellybutton in as you put your arms between your legs and grab your ankles or the lower halves of your legs, with your thumbs on the inside and your fingers on the outside.

- *Imagine you are a grizzly bear playfully stretching in the grass as you lift your feet off the ground and extend your legs wide.* **Photo A**

- Come out of the balance with your legs bent and your toes on the mat.

- Repeat 2 more times.

A

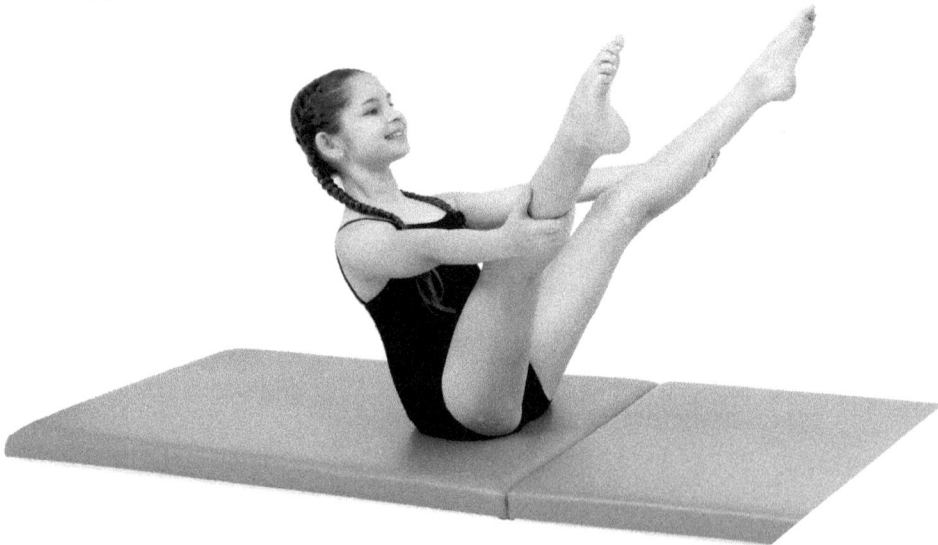

Deeper Practice

- Extend your legs to the top front corners of the room and hold your balance for three counts. **Photo A**

- Scoop out your stomach muscles even deeper as you draw your straight legs together in front of you while keeping your legs elevated above the mat. Hold this balance for an additional three counts. **Photo B**

- Open your legs out to the top front corners of the room and balance for three more counts before returning to starting position with your toes touching each other on the mat.

B

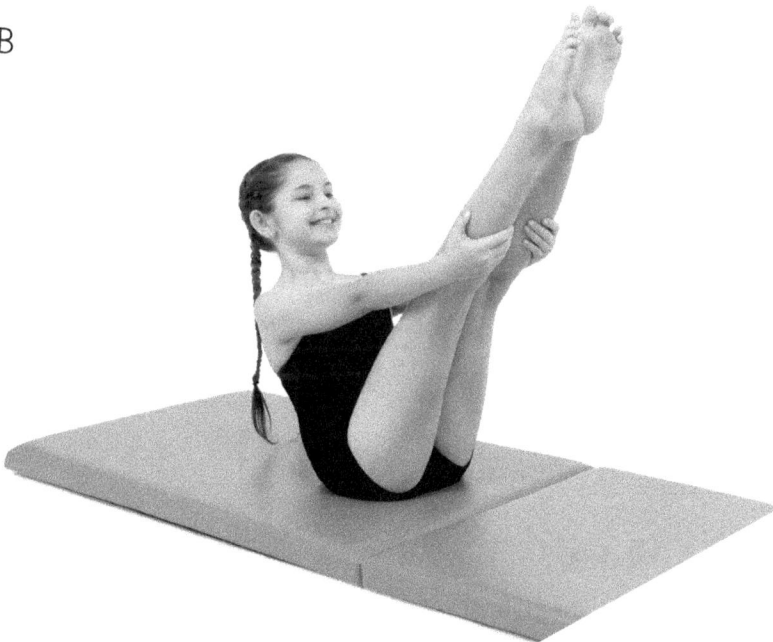

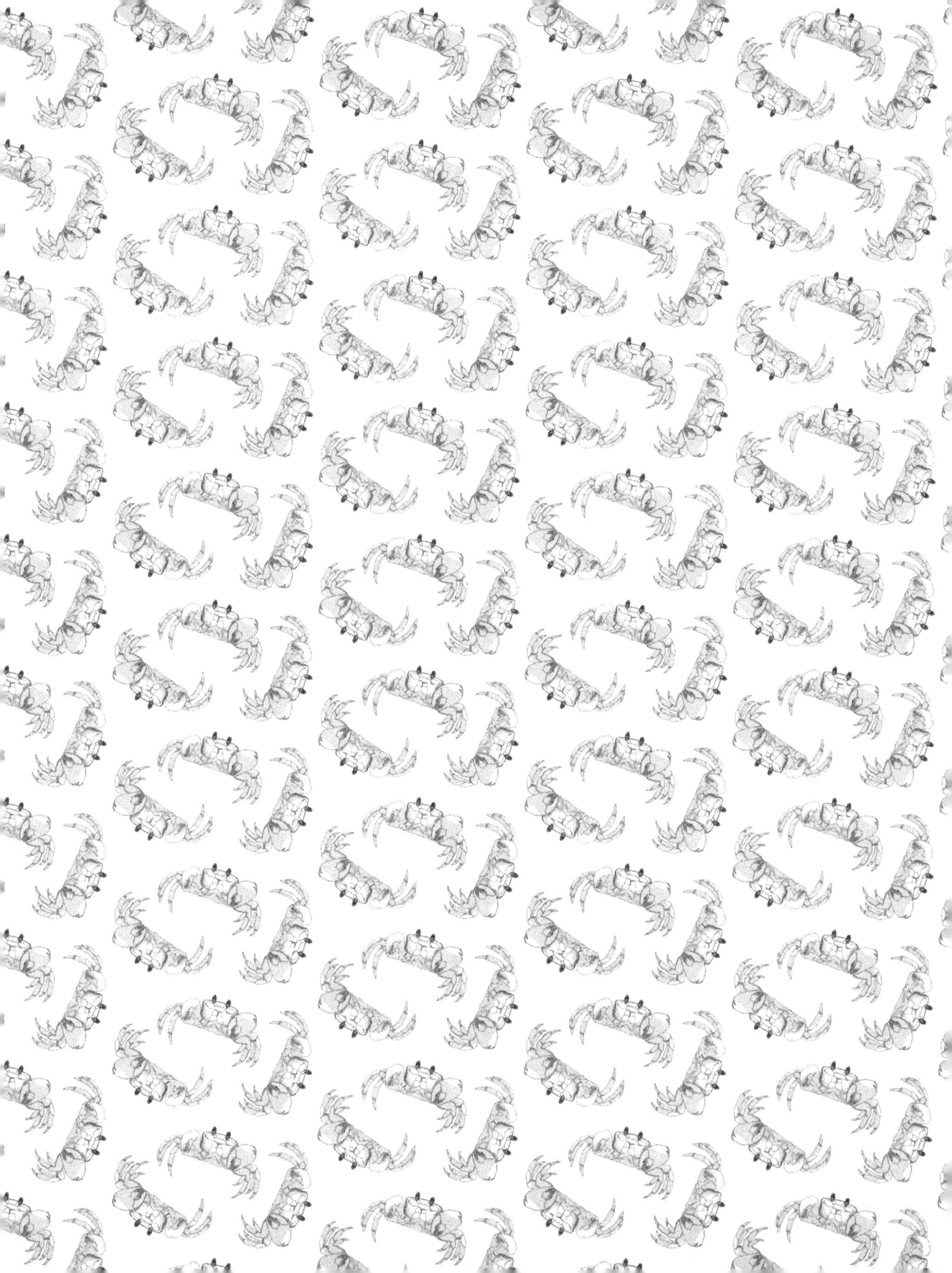

Crab

Crabs are called decapods because they have ten legs, but the front two legs are claws that are rarely used for locomotion. Many crabs can actually shuffle slowly forward, but because their legs are on the sides of their bodies and their leg joints bend outward, crabs move much faster by walking sideways.

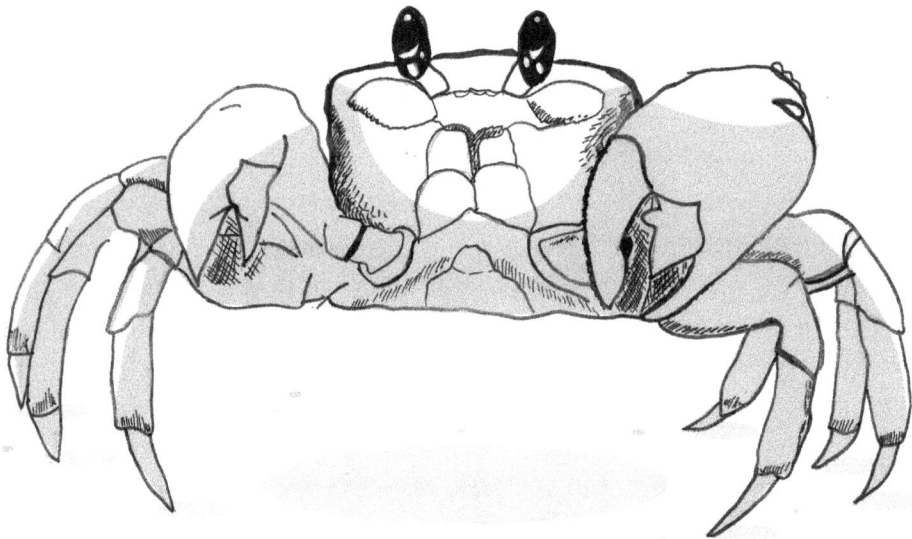

Crawling Crab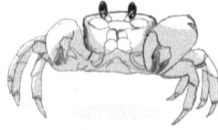

Starting Out

- Bend your knees and place your feet parallel and apart in front of you on the floor.
- Put your hands behind you on the mat with fingertips pointing toward you.
- Lift your hips and hold your shape for 3-10 seconds. **Photo A**
- Perform 3 times.

A

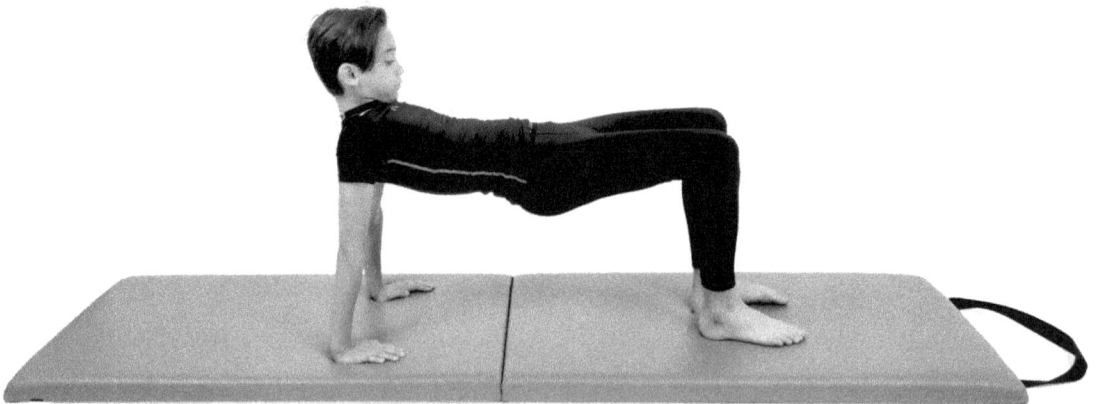

Deeper Practice

- Go into the tabletop shape. **Photo A**

- Walk your hands and feet forward, then backward, while keeping your seat muscles active and your hips lifted. **Photo B**

- You can also walk your hands and feet to one side and then to the other side. *Imagine you are scuttling sideways like a crab.*

B

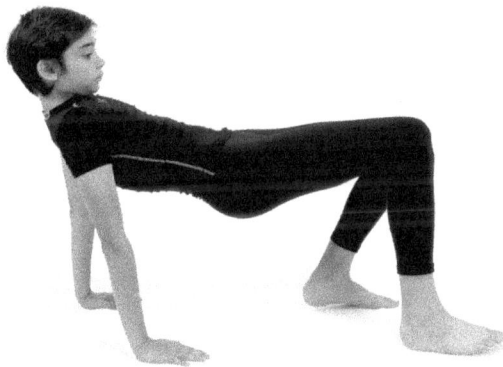

Monkey

Monkeys often scratch their armpits as a means of expressing joy. Like humans, monkeys peel their bananas and do not eat the skins, but unlike us, they peel their bananas from the bottom and use the stem as a handle.

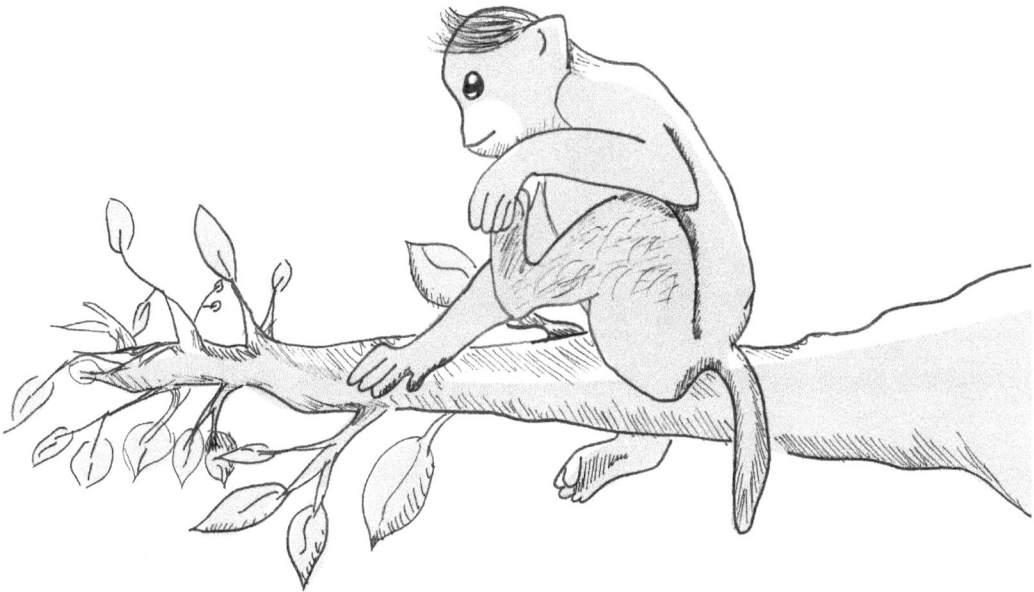

Monkey Business

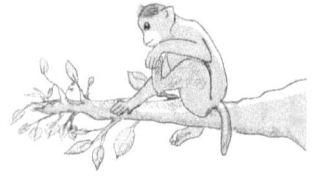

Starting Out

- Sit with your feet and legs together, slightly bent.

- Put a small towel under your heels and hold the towel at each end. **Photo A**

- Holding the towel, slide your heels forward and bend your body forward over your legs. **Photo B**

- Breathe out on the stretch and hold the stretch for only three seconds.

- Slide your heels back into starting position to sit tall.

- Perform 3 times.

A

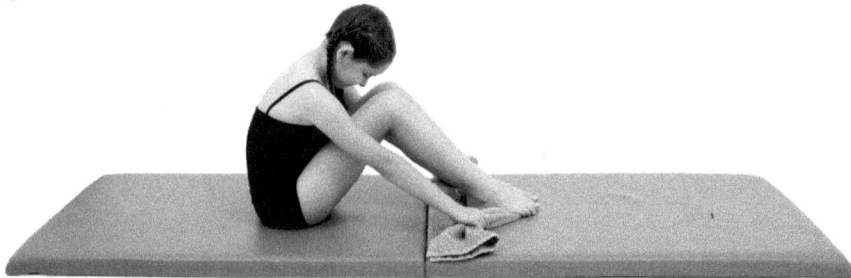

B

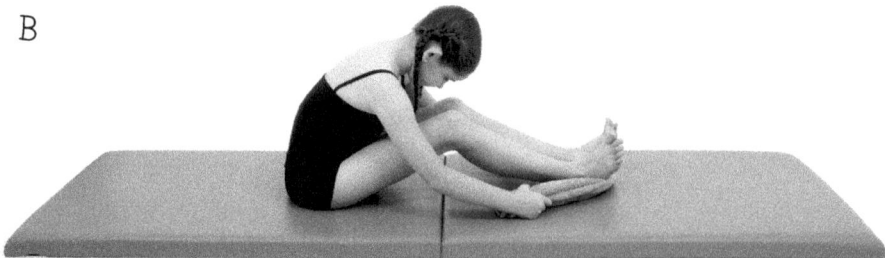

Deeper Practice

- Begin seated, legs together and knees slightly bent.
- Slide your fingertips up the sides of your body as you pull up tall. **Photo C**
- Next, let your fingertips "drip" down the sides of your body, toward the floor, and out toward your toes.
- *As you grab your toes, imagine that you are a monkey reaching for bananas on a tree.*
- With your fingertips holding your toes, slide your heels forward, stretching your legs to the best of your ability as you breathe out for three seconds. **Photo D**
- Slide your heels back into starting position to sit tall.
- Perform 3 times.

C

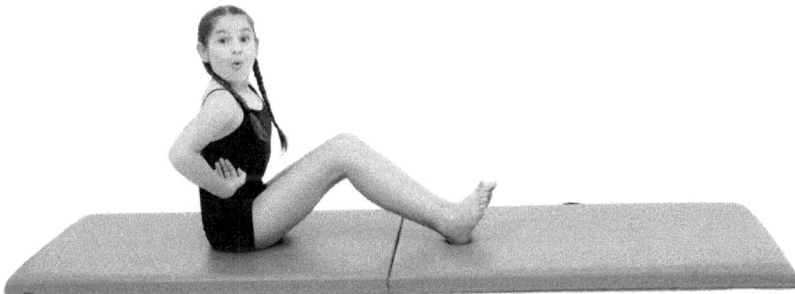

D

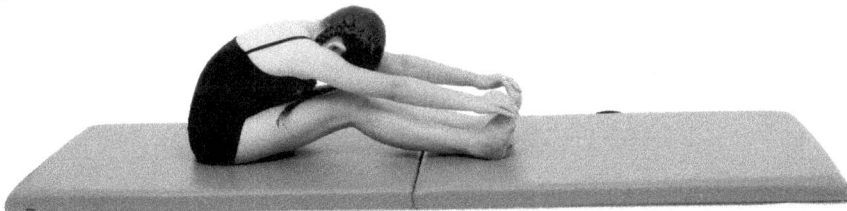

Penguin

Penguins do not fly. Their wings are actually flippers for swimming. Although they are excellent swimmers, their locomotion on land looks a little awkward. Penguins have developed a waddle to compensate for their large webbed feet and for their short legs, set far back on their bodies.

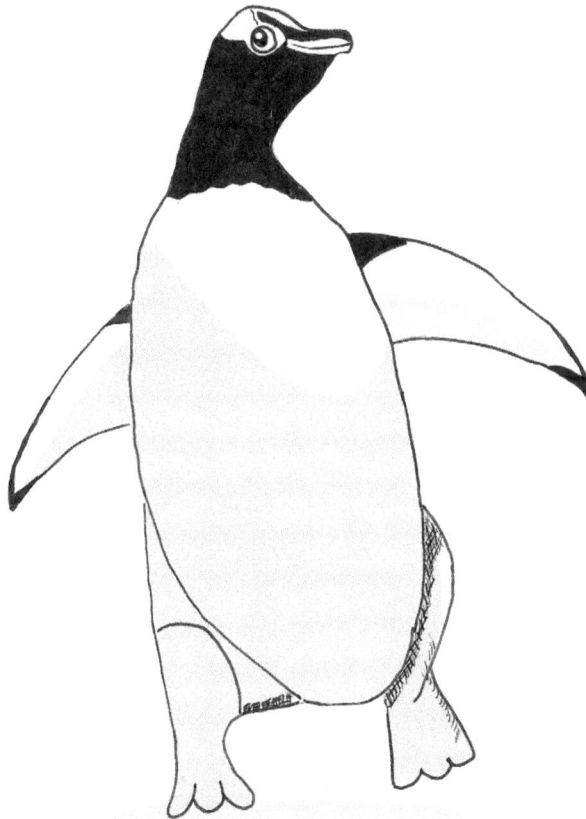

Penguin Waddle

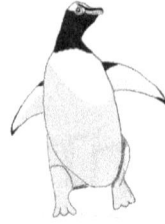

Starting Out

- Sit as tall as you can with your legs stretched out in front of you.

- Stack your forearms and lift your elbows.

- *Pretend that your sitting bones are penguin feet waddling forward as you alternate lifting your sit bones forward in a walking motion.* **Photo A**

- Remember to stay tall in your torso as you move forward.

Deeper Practice

- Once you have the coordination in the forward direction, try to waddle on your "penguin feet" in the reverse direction.

A

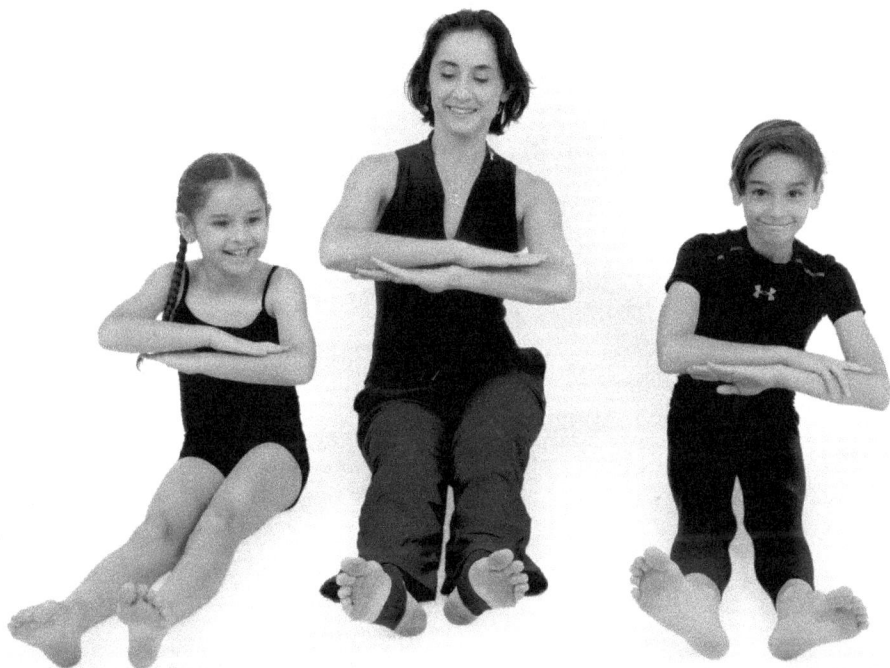

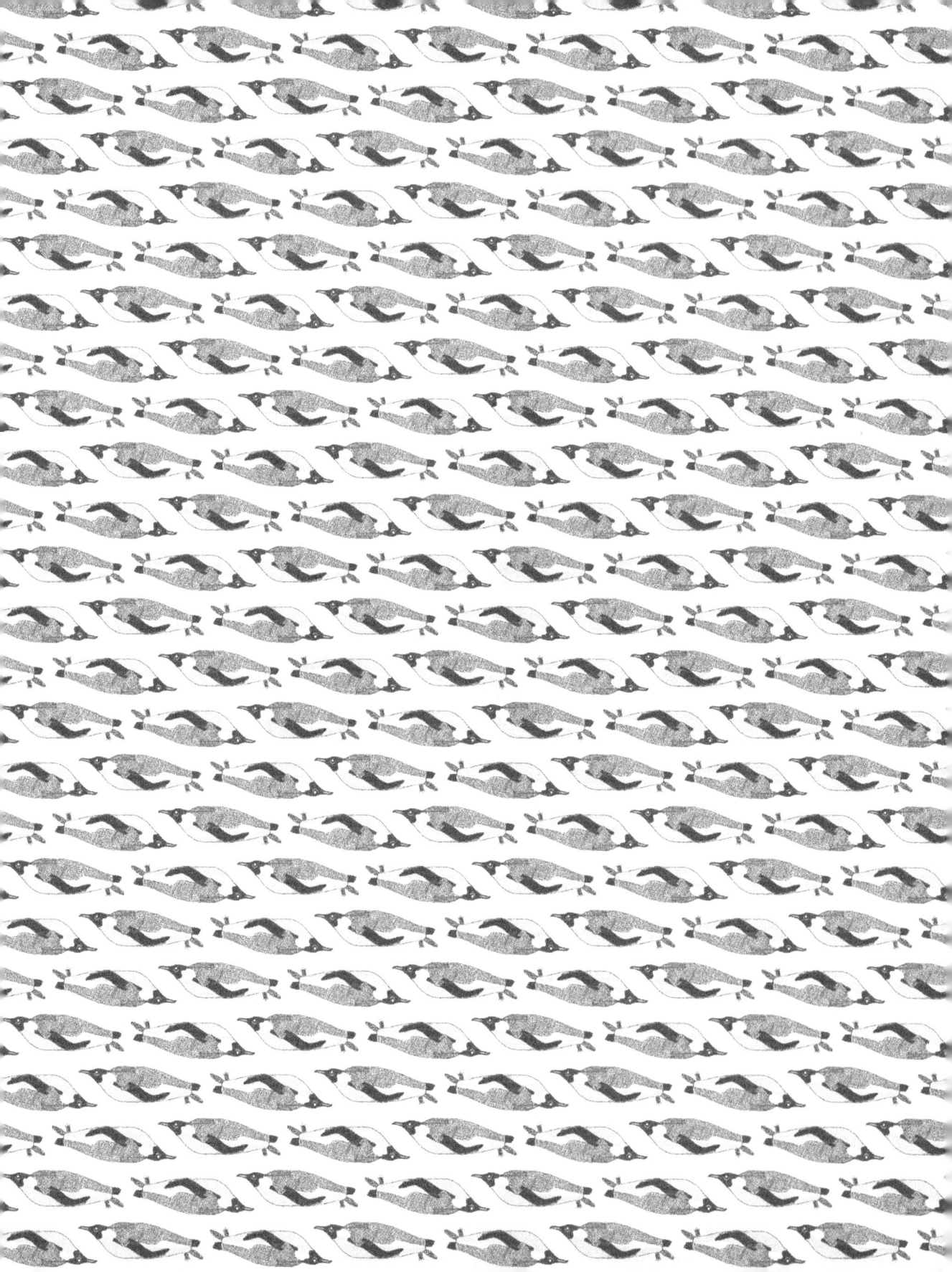

Penguin

Since waddling on land is time consuming, penguins like to slide on their bellies over ice and snow to move faster. This is called tobogganing. This gets them to their destination faster, but penguins also like to slide on their bellies because it's fun.

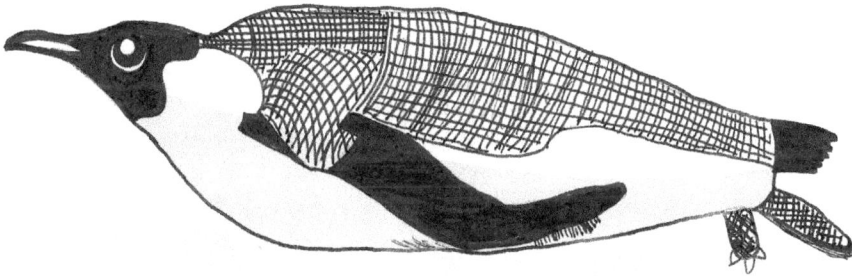

Penguin Belly Slide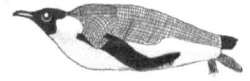

Starting Out

- Lie on your stomach with your head turned to the side, one ear resting on the mat.

- *Your arms are long by your sides like the flippers of a penguin.*

- As you breathe in, turn your face toward the mat and begin to lift your chest.

- You can have a helper gently press on your feet to help you keep your legs on the mat. **Photo A**

- If necessary, you can keep your legs slightly apart.

- As you breathe out, lower your chest and place your other ear on the mat.

- Perform 4 times.

A

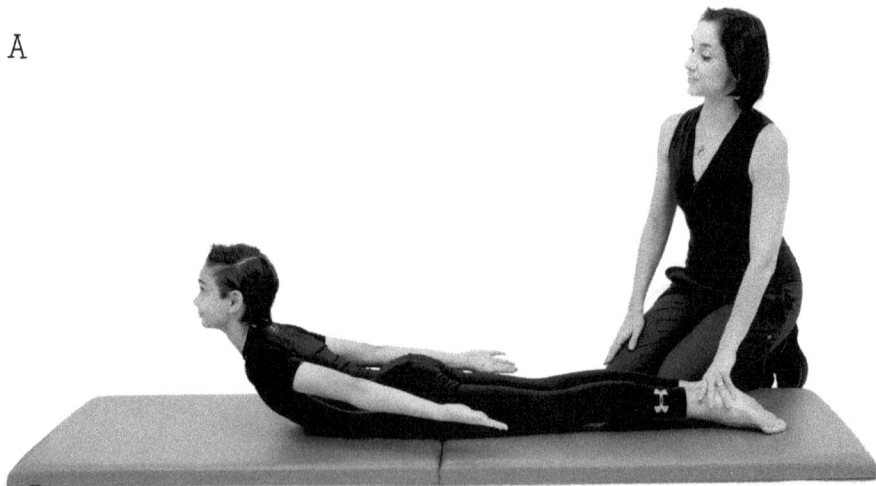

Deeper Practice

- For an added challenge, do the Penguin Belly Slide with your legs tightly together on the mat and without anyone holding your feet. **Photo B**

B

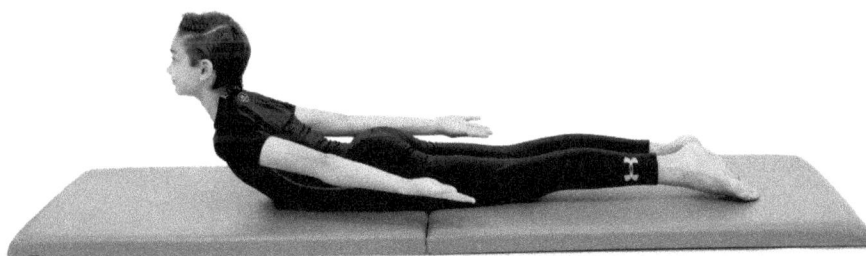

Cricket

When you hear crickets chirping at night you are listening to male crickets sing. The main reason male crickets chirp is to attract the attention of female crickets. The left wing of a male cricket has many ridges and is called the file. The top part of the right wing is the scraper. The file rubbing against the scraper is called stridulation and produces a chirping sound.

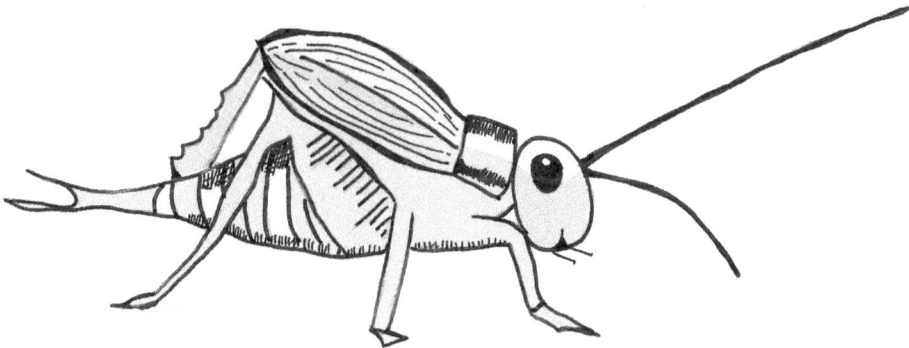

Cricket Wings

Starting Out

- Lie on your stomach and rest your forehead on your stacked hands.
- Remember to pull your bellybutton away from the mat to keep pressure out of your low back.
- Lift your extended legs slightly above the mat.
- Click your heels together 10 times, then rest your legs on the mat. **Photo A**
- Repeat 2 more sets of ten heel beats, taking a rest between each set.

Deeper Practice

- For an added challenge, coordinate the clicking of your heels with a specific breathing sequence. Breathe in for five heel clicks, and breathe out for five heel clicks.
- *Imagine that your legs are the two forewings of a cricket opening and closing simultaneously to produce a song.*
- Repeat 2 more sets.

A

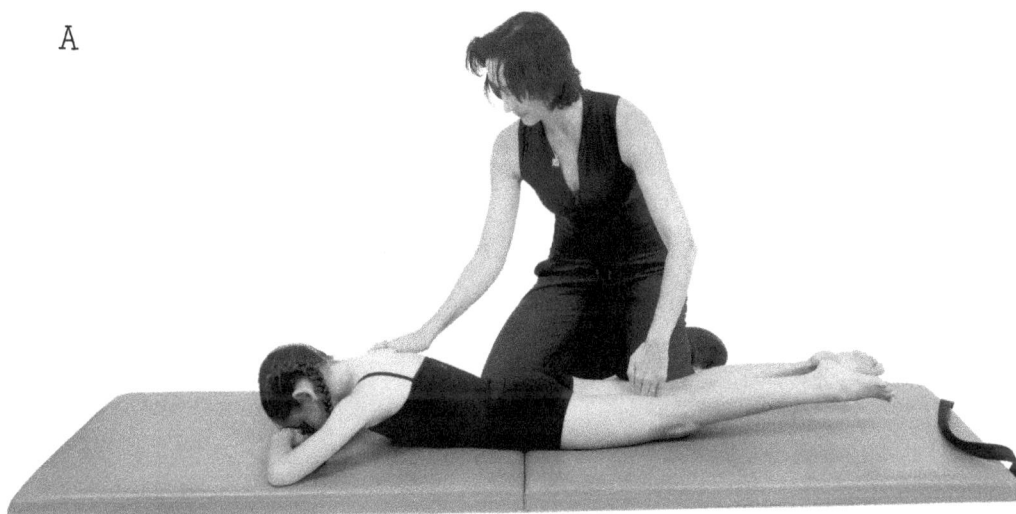

Swan

Swans have long, graceful necks. A male swan is called a cob and a female swan is called a pen. A swan couple stays together for life and shows affection by touching beaks.

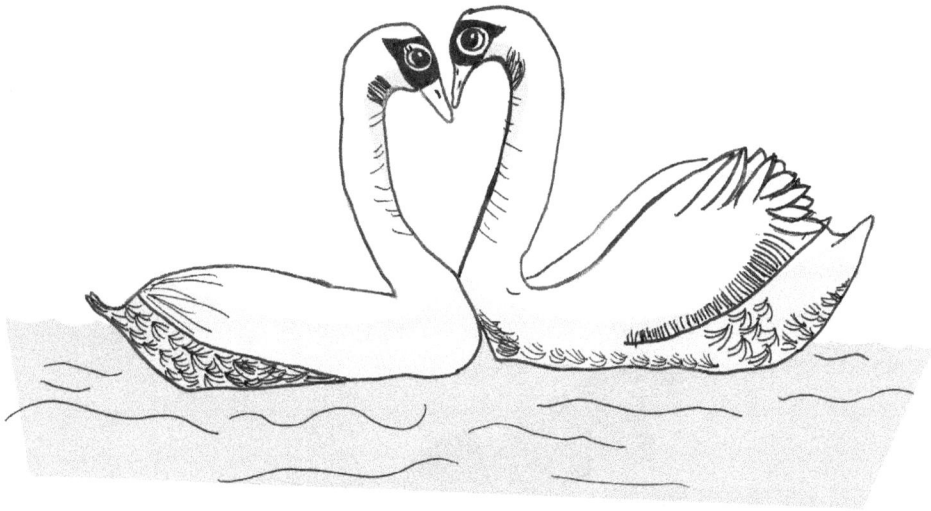

Swan Neck

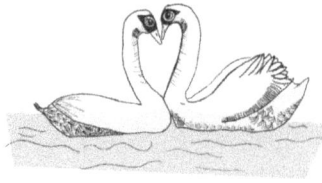

Starting Out

- Lie on your stomach and prop yourself on your elbows.

- Your elbows can be directly under your shoulders with your upper arms perpendicular to the mat, or you can put your elbows forward slightly for a milder stretch.

- *To create the longest and most graceful swan neck possible, and to avoid sinking into the shoulder joints, imagine that someone is lifting you up by your ears.*

- Remember to pull your bellybutton away from the mat as you press your forearms into the mat. **Photo A**

A

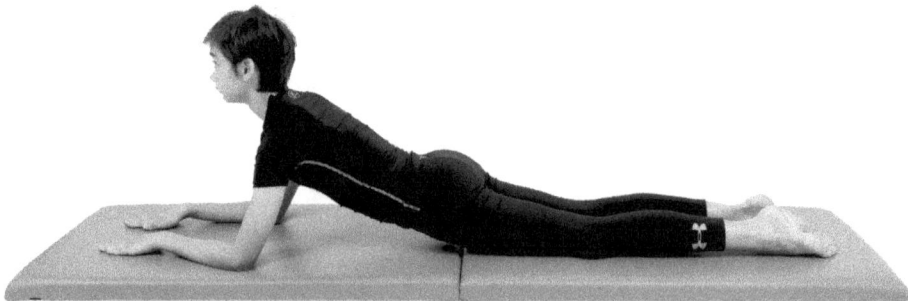

Deeper Practice

- As you get stronger, you can intensify the lift in your chest by straightening your arms: leave your hands on the mat, lift your elbows off the mat, and pull yourself forward and up. **Photo B**

B

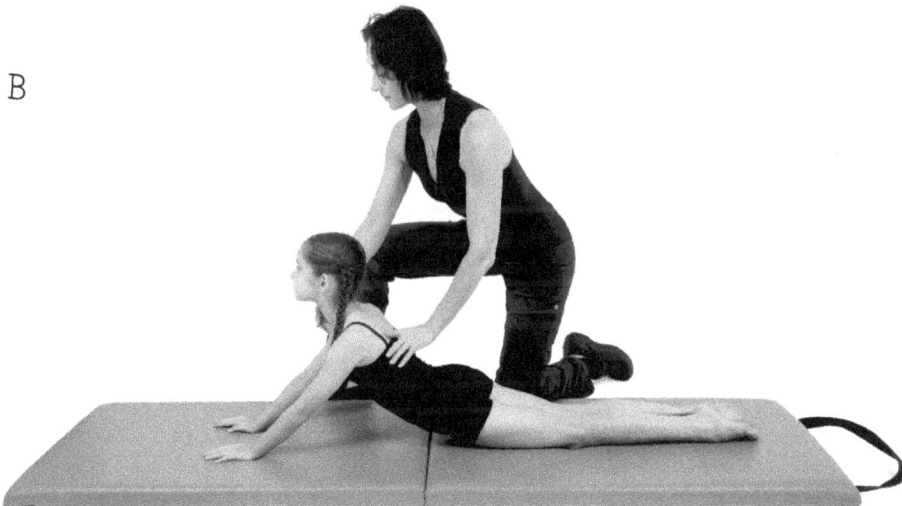

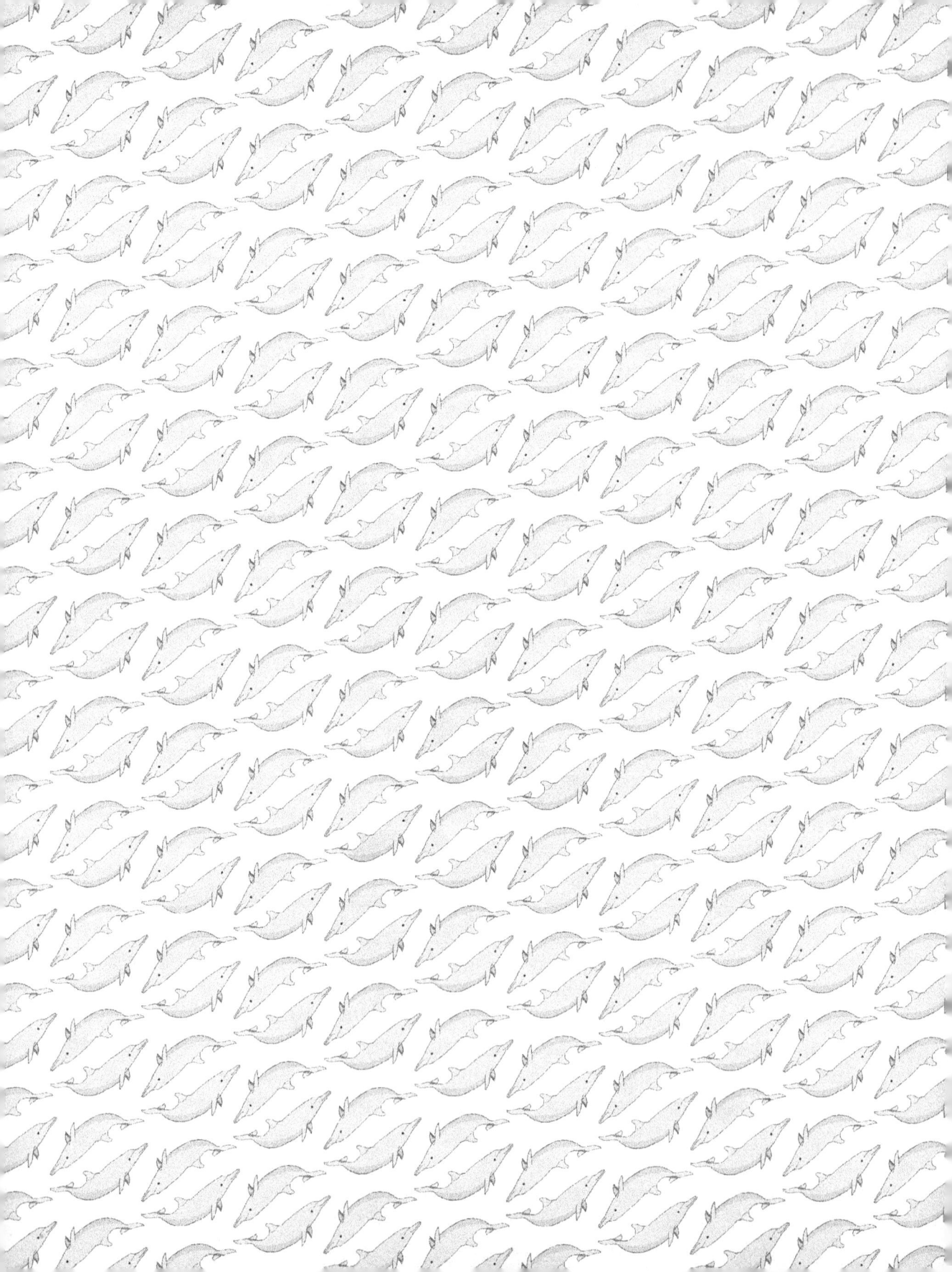

Dolphin

A dolphin's smooth and streamlined body helps make it a very fast swimmer, but it is the dolphin's tail, or fluke, that gives it its power. Unlike most fish that move their tails side to side as they swim, the dolphin moves its tail fluke up and down to move forward.

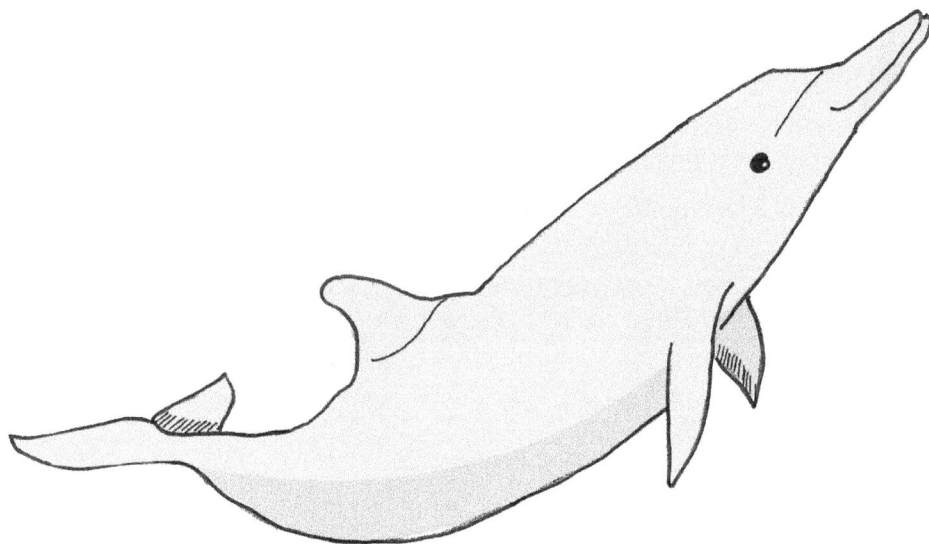

Dolphin Tail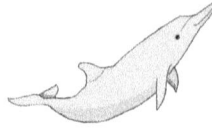

Starting Out

- Begin lying on your stomach with your forehead resting on your hands and your legs stretched.

- With your stomach pulled in, try to lift your knees above the mat keeping your legs straight. **Photo A**

- Keep your knees above the mat and slowly bend them, bringing your feet toward your seat. **Photo B**

Deeper Practice

- When you are ready to build on the first sequence, pulse your heels toward your seat three times before stretching your legs back out on the mat.

- To keep your low back protected, you must keep your abdominals active.

- *As you pulse your heels, imagine that your legs are the tail fluke of a dolphin moving up and down as you swim forward.*

- Perform 4 sets of 3 heel pulses.

A

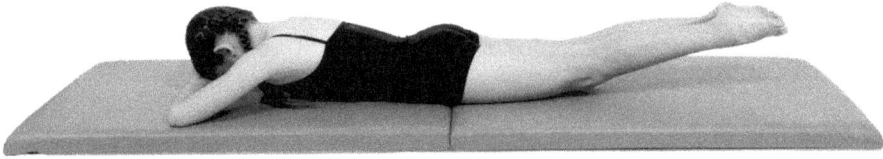

B

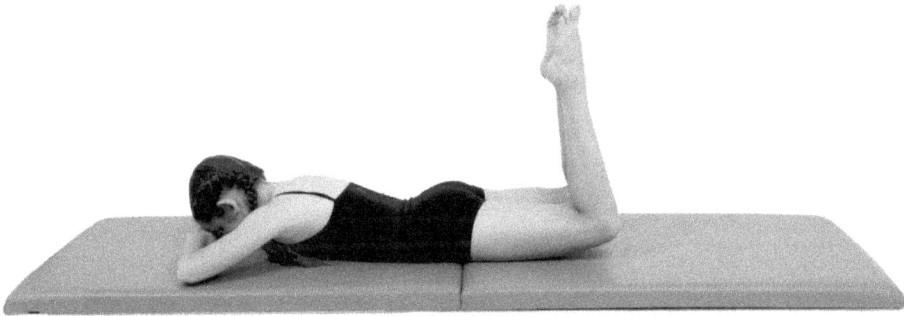

Seal

Although seals are very fast in the water, their inability to rotate their hind flippers make them belly crawlers on land. They are often seen propped up on their front set of flippers with their hind flippers raised.

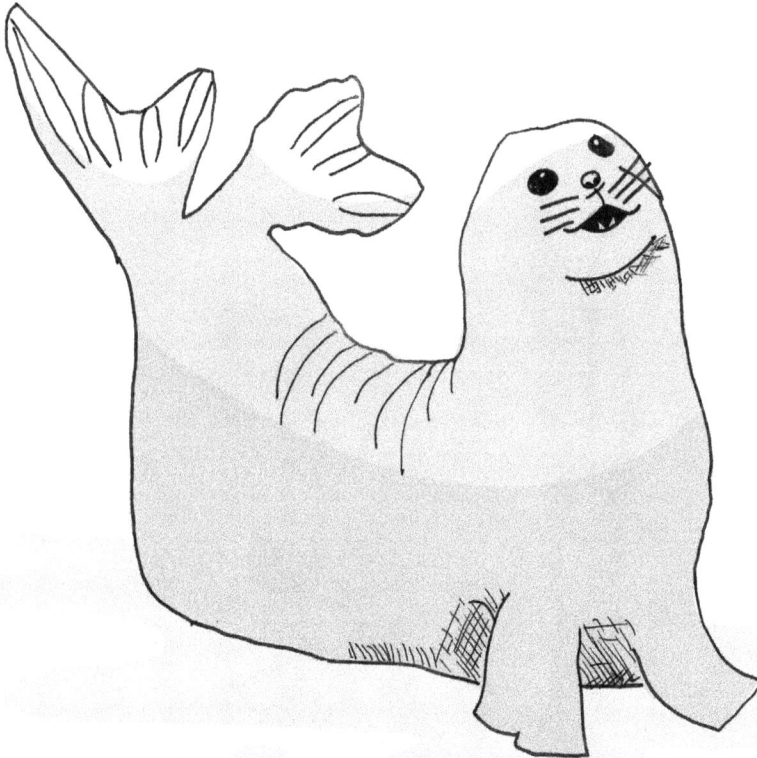

Hungry Seal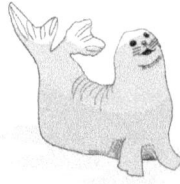

Starting Out

- Lie on your stomach and position your hands shoulder width apart on the mat. Your hands are under your shoulders, or farther forward for a slightly milder stretch.

- With your stomach muscles pulled in, push your hands into the mat as you lift your chest.

- *As you bend your knees, bringing your toes toward your head, imagine you are a seal raising your hind flippers.* **Photo A**

- Hold the position up to three seconds, then rest.

- Perform up to 3 times.

A

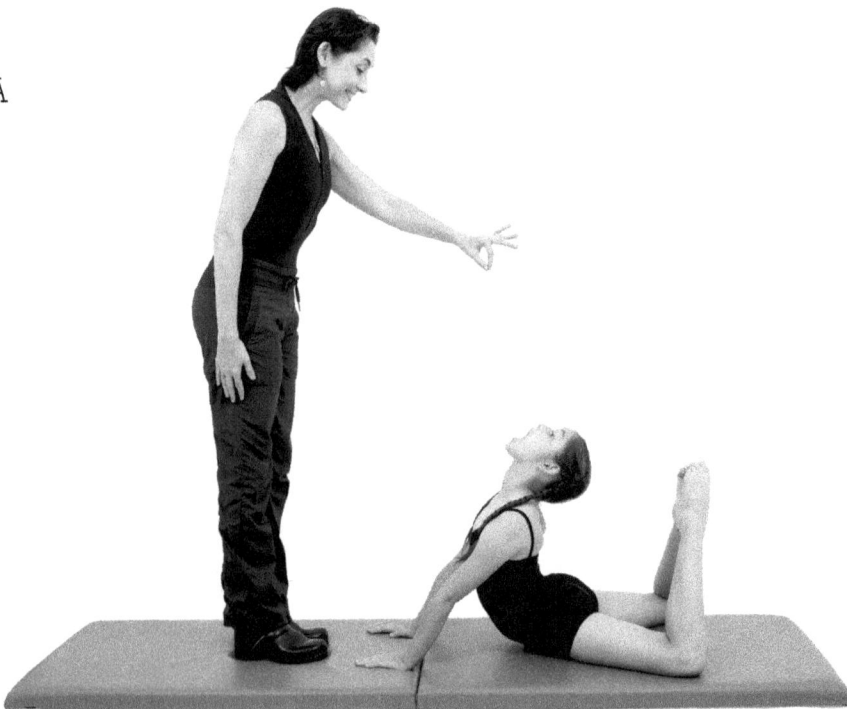

Deeper Practice

- Bend your knees while lying on your stomach and grab the tops of your feet.

- Lift your chest and thighs.

- Push the tops of your feet into your hands to facilitate the lift in your body. **Photo B**

- Hold the position up to three seconds.

- Perform up to 3 times.

B

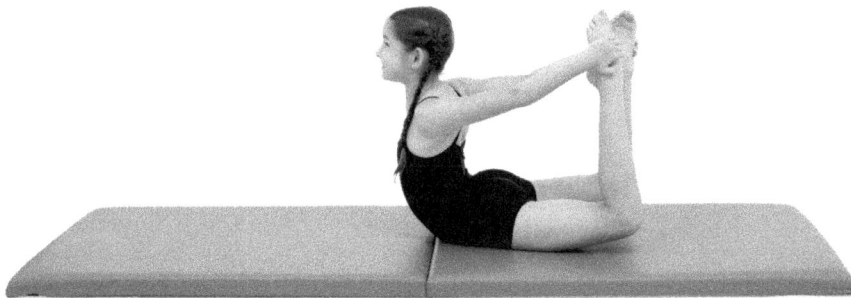

Beetle

Ladybugs are a kind of beetle. They have a round, protective shell, which hides the delicate pair of flying wings that lie underneath the hard pair of wings when the ladybug is not flying.

Ladybugs are extremely helpful in the garden because they eat bugs that are harmful to plants. To help defend themselves from predators, ladybugs play dead. They can also emit a yellow fluid that other bugs find unappealing.

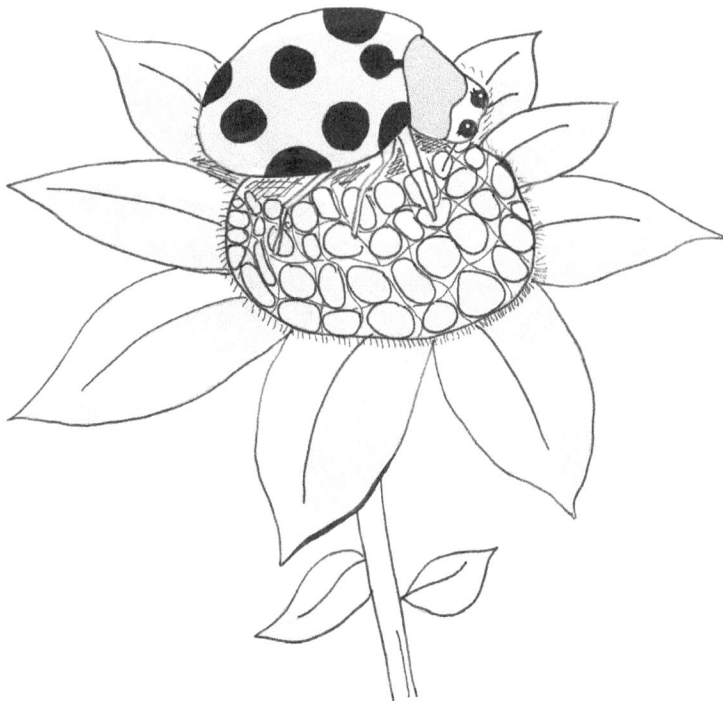

Beetle Wings

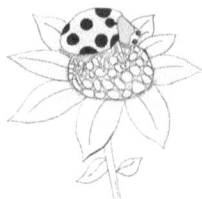

Starting Out

- Kneel and sit back on your heels.

- Your arms stretch back toward your toes with your palms facing the ceiling.

- To maximize the stretch in your low back, round your back without letting your head touch the mat. **Photo A**

A

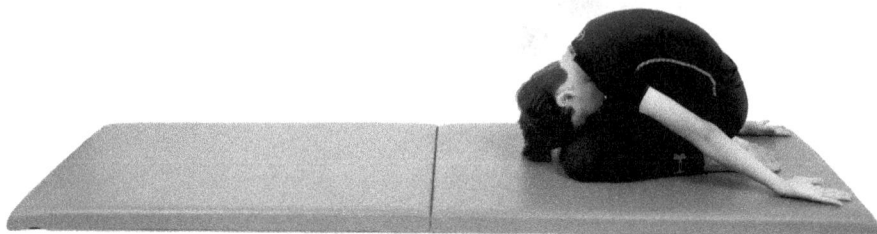

Deeper Practice

- *As you sit back on your heels kneeling, imagine you are a beetle with a round, protective shell.*

- To stretch your toe joints, curl your toes under, toes pointing toward your knees.

- To deepen the stretch in your low back, grab the soles of your feet and pull them gently as you pull your stomach in. **Photo B**

B

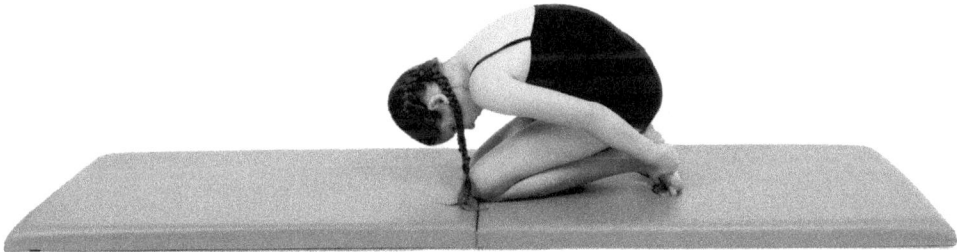

Dog

A happy dog usually wants to play, and one of the ways she expresses this is by sticking her rear end up in the air while she lowers her chest and lifts her gaze. This is called a play bow.

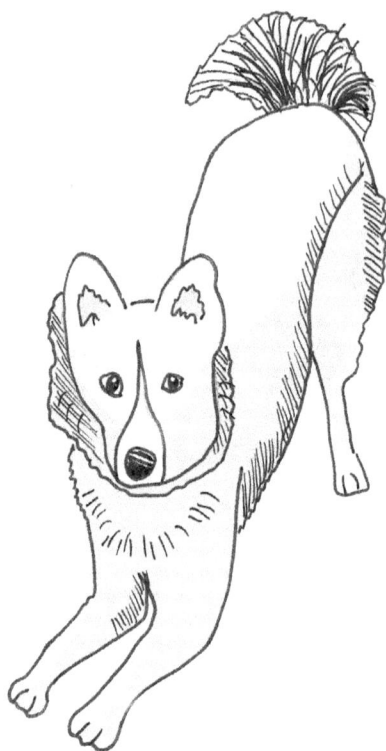

Cat

Joe Pilates liked to watch the movement of cats because they are always stretching. Part of the reason their spines are so flexible is that they have about double the amount of vertebrae we have. When a cat is frightened, he will try to make himself threatening by appearing bigger to his opponent. He rounds his back into a half moon shape and if he is very frightened, the fur on his back and tail will stick out on end, making him look even bigger.

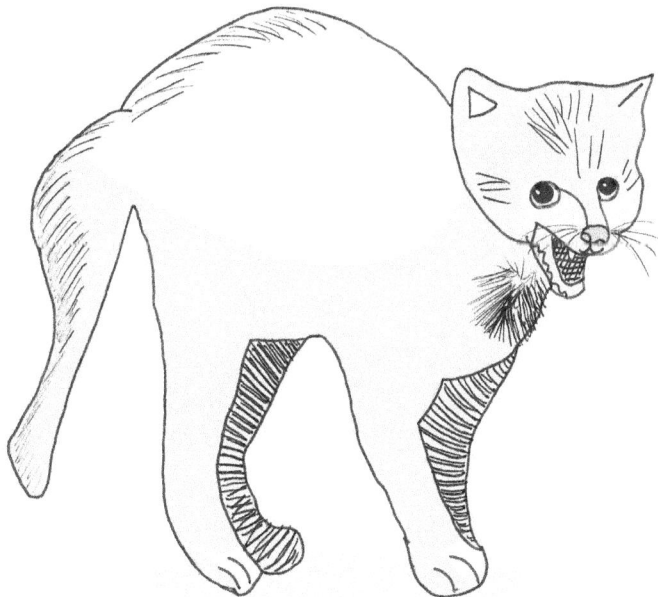

Happy Dog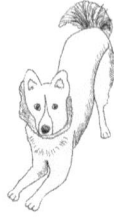

- Kneel with your feet and legs apart, and your hands on the mat, shoulder width apart.
- Your hips are above your knees and your shoulders are directly above your hands.
- Pull your stomach muscles in as you stick your seat out slightly and lift your head. *Imagine you are a playful dog.* **Photo A**
- Note: The Happy Dog exercise should be performed together with the Angry Cat exercise.

A

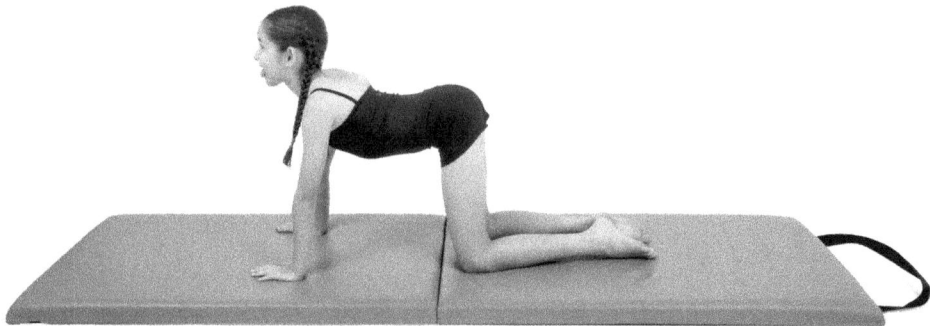

Angry Cat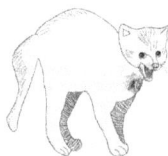

- From the Happy Dog shape, round your back into a half moon as you lower your head and look toward your bellybutton. *Imagine you are a frightened cat.*
- To deepen the stretch in your low back, push the floor away with your hands as you lift your waist. **Photo B**
- Alternate arching the back in the Happy Dog shape and rounding the back in the Angry Cat shape several times. Always finish with the rounded back.

B

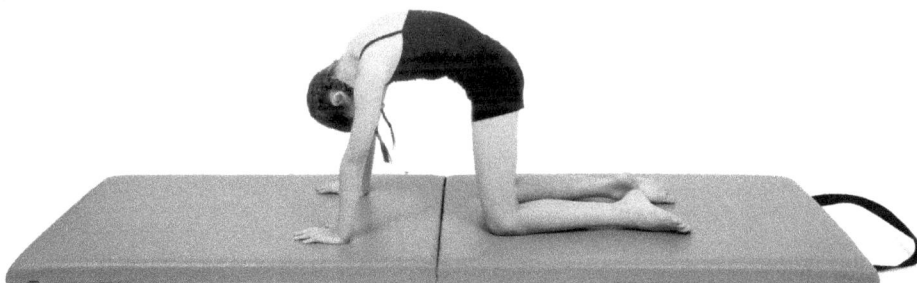

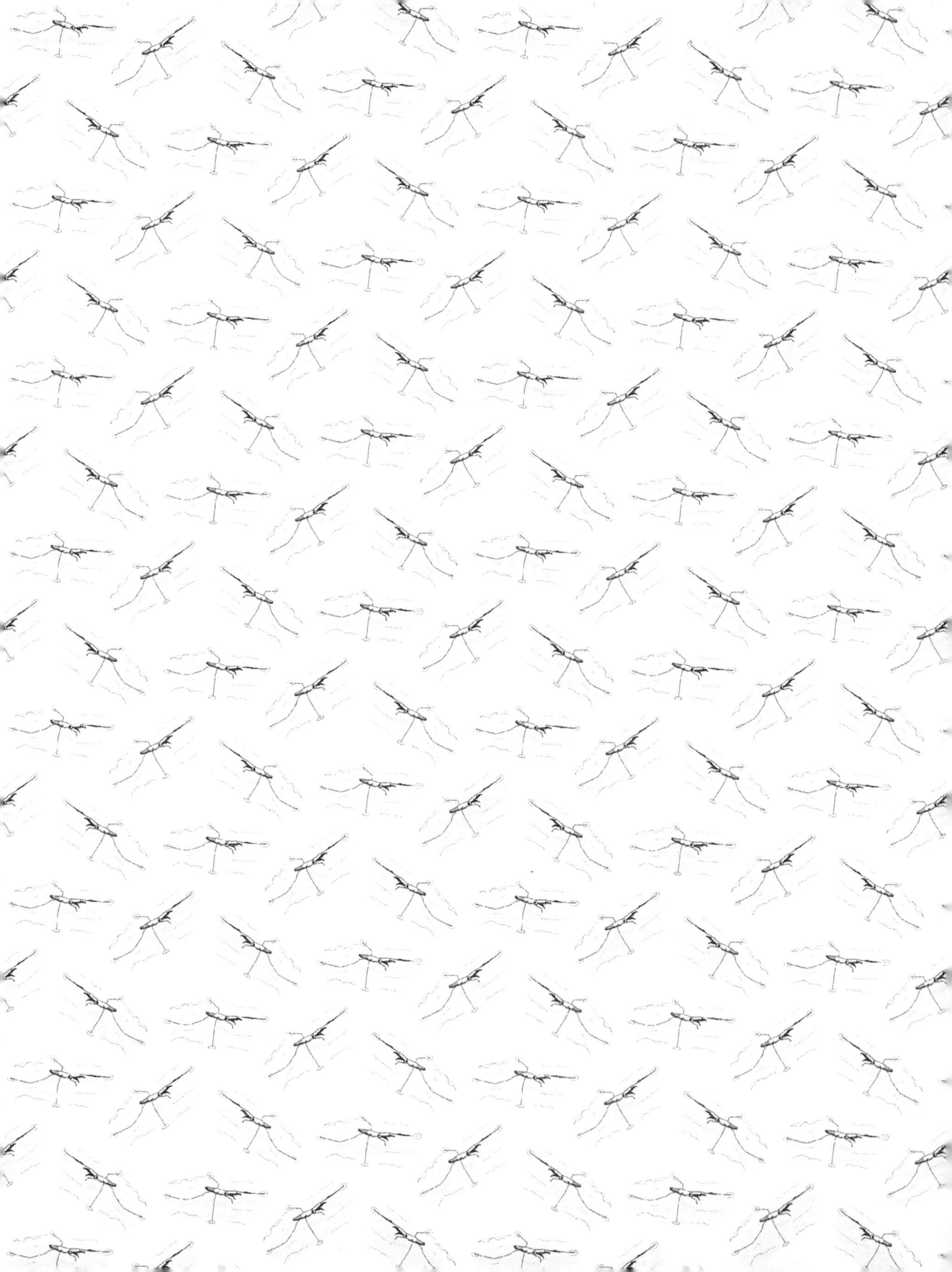

Water Strider

A water strider is a bug usually found in freshwater ponds and lakes. It can glide on the surface of the water by distributing its weight evenly among its four long legs in the back and middle, and two shorter legs in the front. The legs have tiny hairs that repel water and capture air. The air allows the water strider to float easily over the surface of the water. It is a very useful insect because it eats mosquitos.

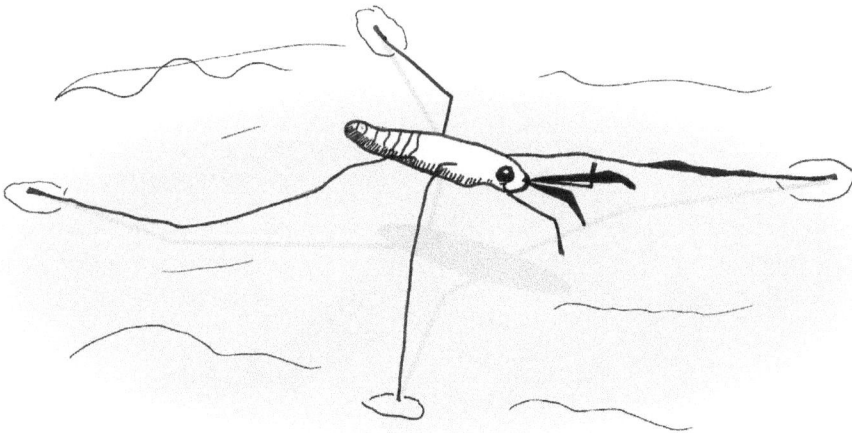

Water Strider

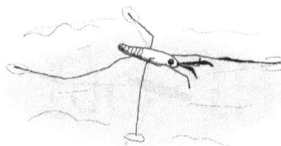

Starting Out

- Kneel with your hips directly above your knees and your shoulders directly above your hands.

- With your toes curled forward, lower your head and round your back.

- Pull your bellybutton away from the floor as your knees lift above the mat, knees level with your heels or slightly higher.

- Keeping the weight mostly in your hands, keep one leg bent with the knee hovering above the mat as you slide your other foot back until your leg stretches behind you. **Photo A**

- As you alternate sliding your feet past each other, make sure not to let your upper body bounce up and down.

- Perform 3-5 sets.

A

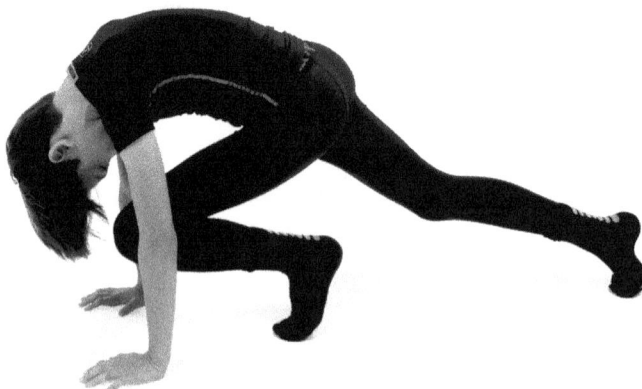

Deeper Practice

- Once you have mastered isolating your torso as your legs slide past each other, you can slide your legs in and out in unison. **Photo B**

- Be sure that your feet remain hip bone width apart throughout the sliding movement, and that your hips and upper body remain isolated from the movement in the legs.

- *Imagine you are a water bug skating on the surface of a pond.*

- Perform 3-5 times.

B

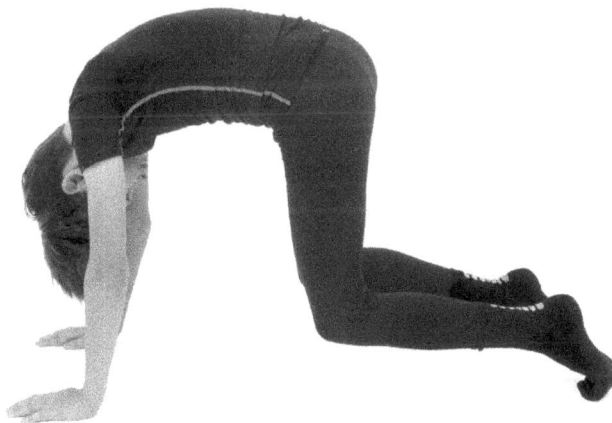

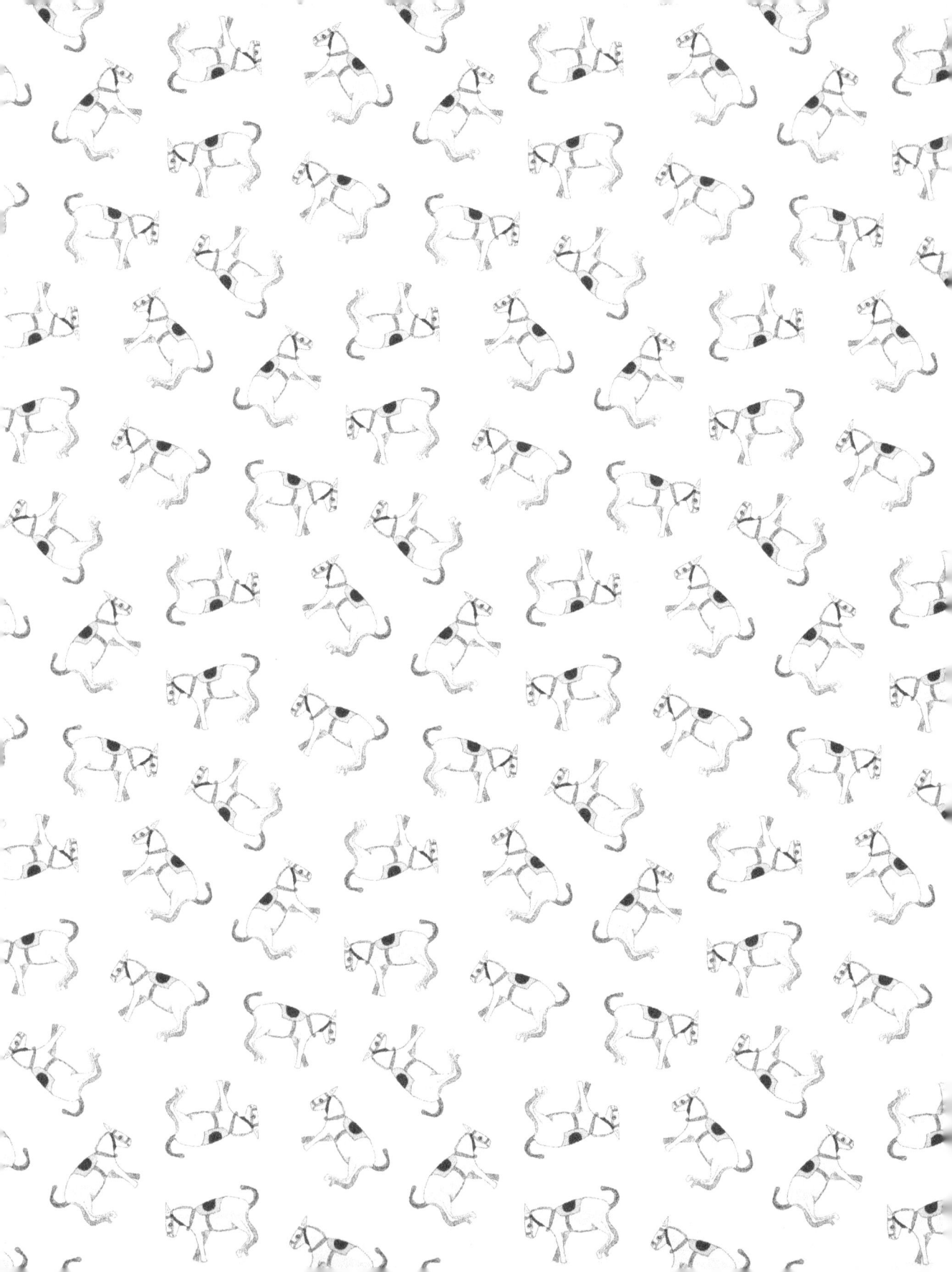

Donkey

Donkeys have an excellent memory and are capable of remembering someone they met up to 25 years earlier. Donkeys get a bad reputation for being stubborn, but in fact it is their intelligence we see when donkeys dig in their heels. Donkeys will not move if they sense there is danger nearby.

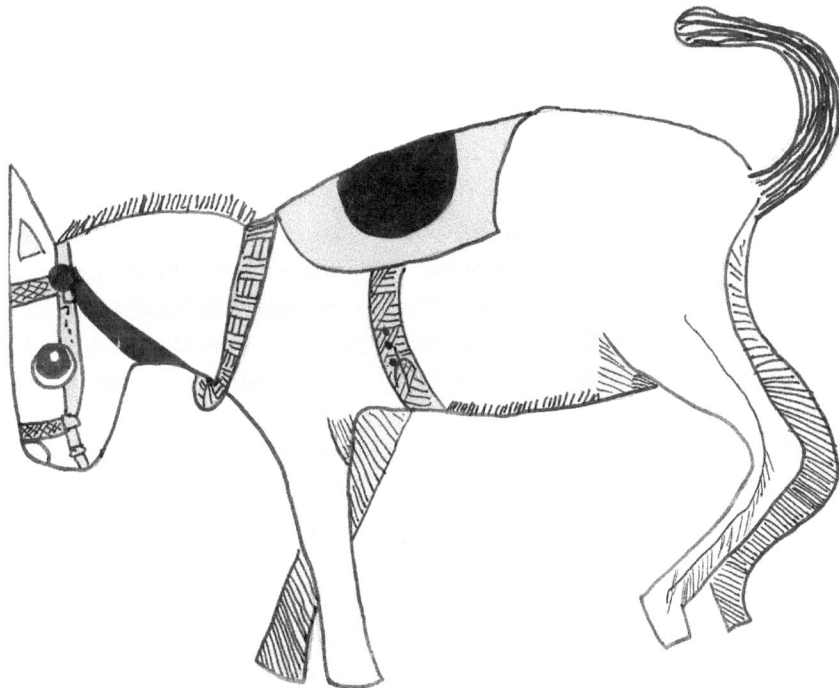

Donkey Kick

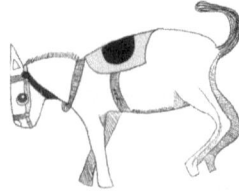

Starting Out

- Kneel with your hips directly above your knees and your shoulders directly above your hands.

- With your waist lifted and head down, lift one leg off the mat and extend it behind you. **Photo A**

- Then bend the same leg toward your nose. **Photo B**

- Alternate stretching and bending your leg 3 times, then repeat the movement on the other side.

- *Imagine that you are a donkey, kicking your hind leg back in an effort to defend yourself.*

- Remember to pull your bellybutton in and to work with control as you move your leg.

A

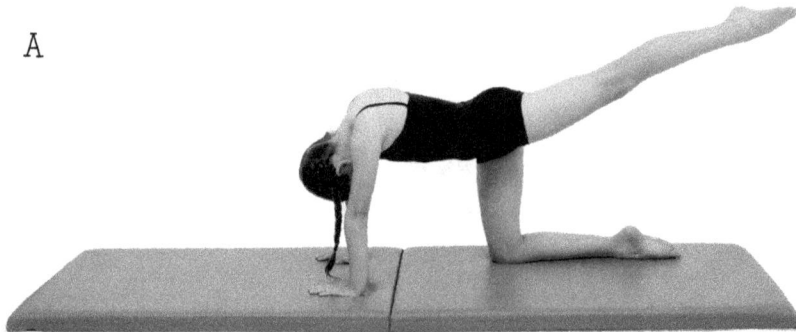

B

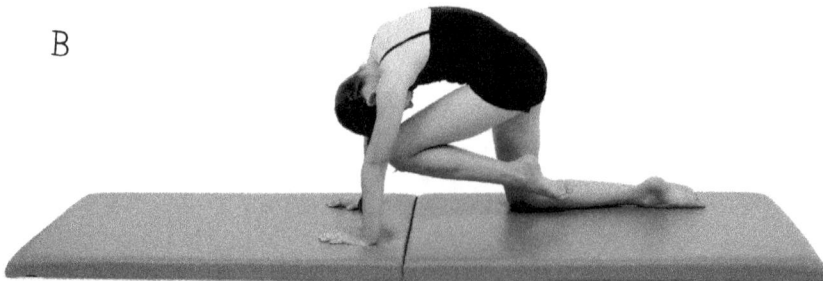

Deeper Practice

- If you are strong enough to support more weight in your hands and toes, you can curl your toes forward and lift your knees off the mat.

- Keep your supporting knee above the mat and isolate your body as your other leg stretches and bends 3 times without touching the mat. **Photos C-D**

- Repeat on the other side.

C

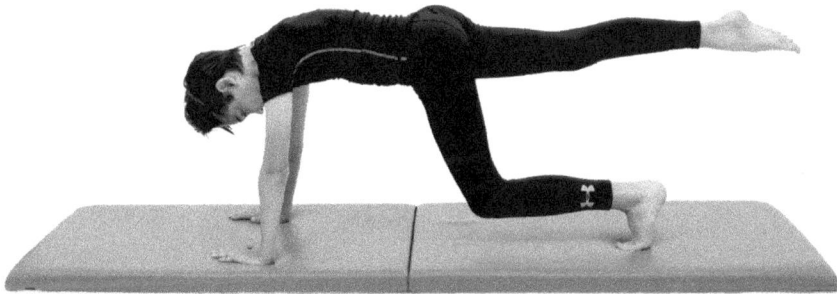

D

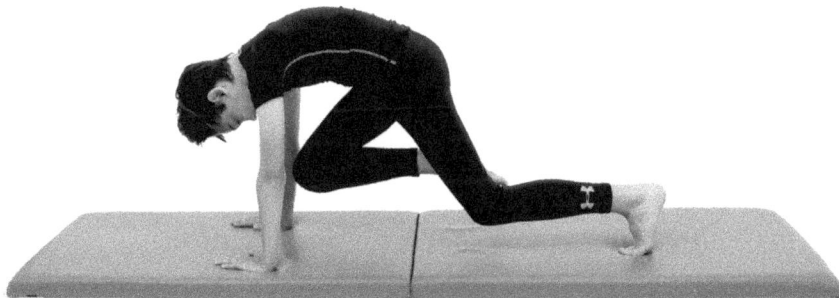

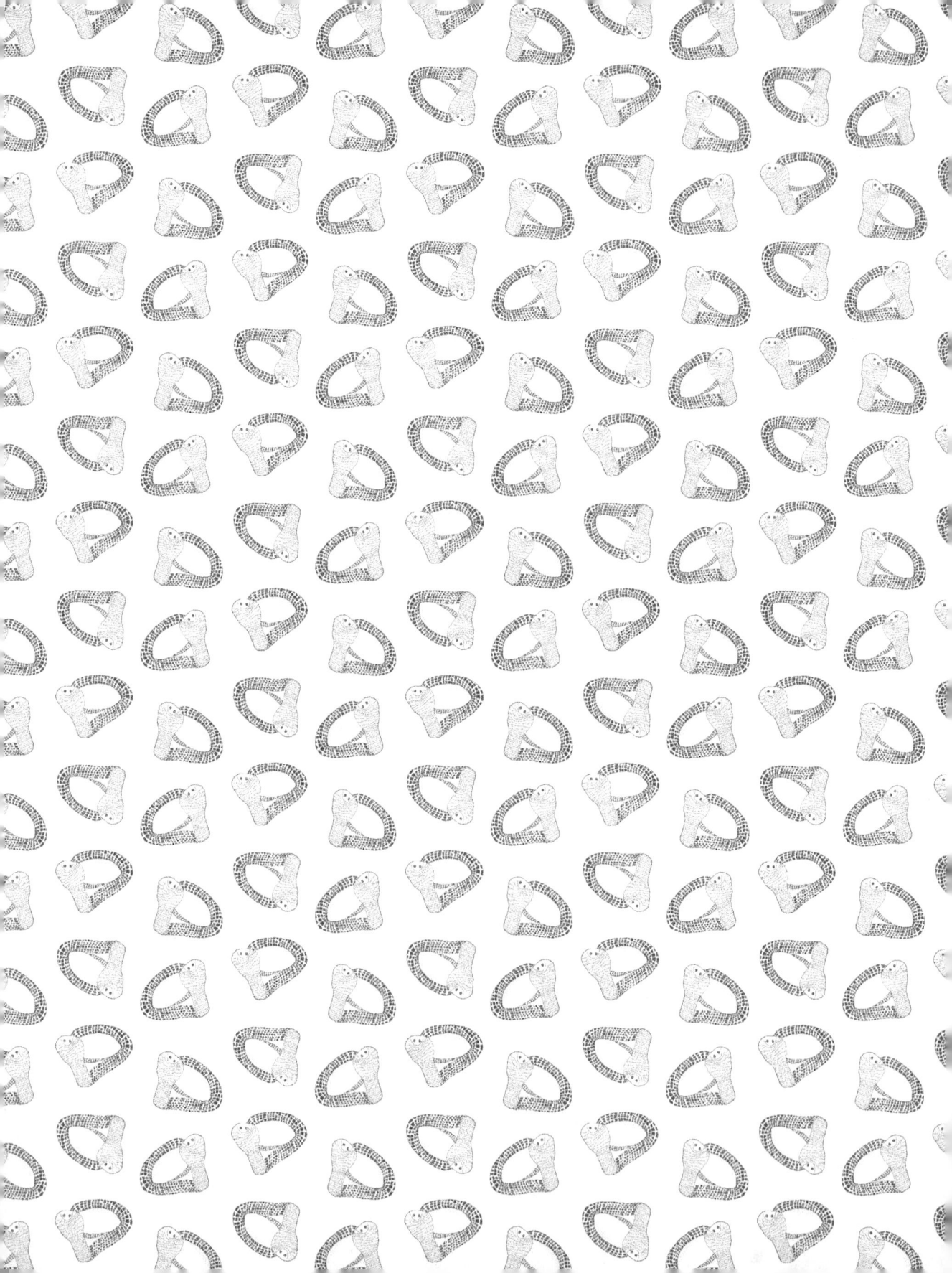

Snake

A snake can lift its head high above the ground when he or she feels threatened by a predator. Just as a frightened cat makes herself look bigger to intimidate her opponent, some snakes, cobras especially, can make a threatening hood at the neck in order to intimidate the opponent.

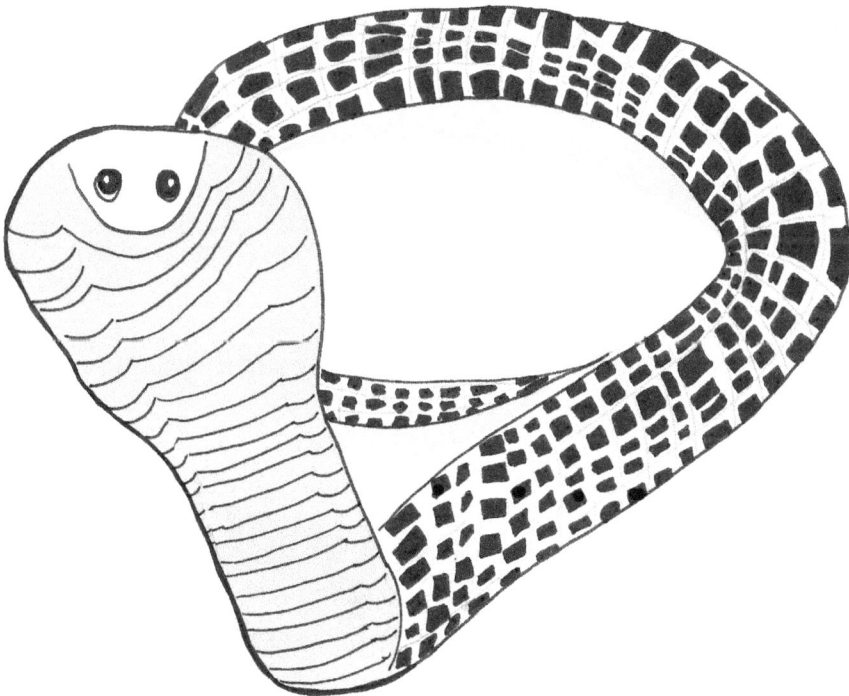

Hissing Snake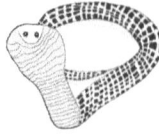

Starting Out

- Kneel with your feet and knees apart and your toes curled under.

- Your hands are on the mat, directly under your shoulders, and your hips are above your knees.

- Take a deep breath and walk your hands forward.

- Then lift your chest and press your hips forward as you breathe out for three counts. **Photo A**

- To avoid collapsing into your low back, pretend that you are pushing the floor away as you lift your bellybutton in and up toward the ceiling.

- Walk your hands back to the starting position to complete the movement.

- Perform 3-5 times.

A

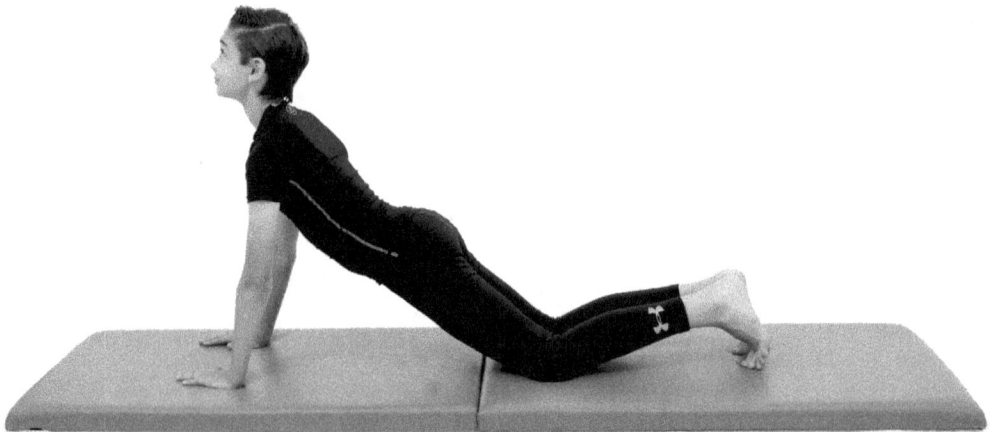

Deeper Practice

- For an extra challenge, try the Hissing Snake with the knees above the mat.

- Stand on all fours with your hips in the air.

- Walk your hands forward, going into a plank shape, then lower your hips slightly as your bellybutton pulls in deeper and your chest lifts. *For fun, you can hiss like a snake as you hold this shape.* **Photo B**

- Lower your head and lift your hips toward the ceiling between repetitions, as a breather.

- Perform 3 times.

B

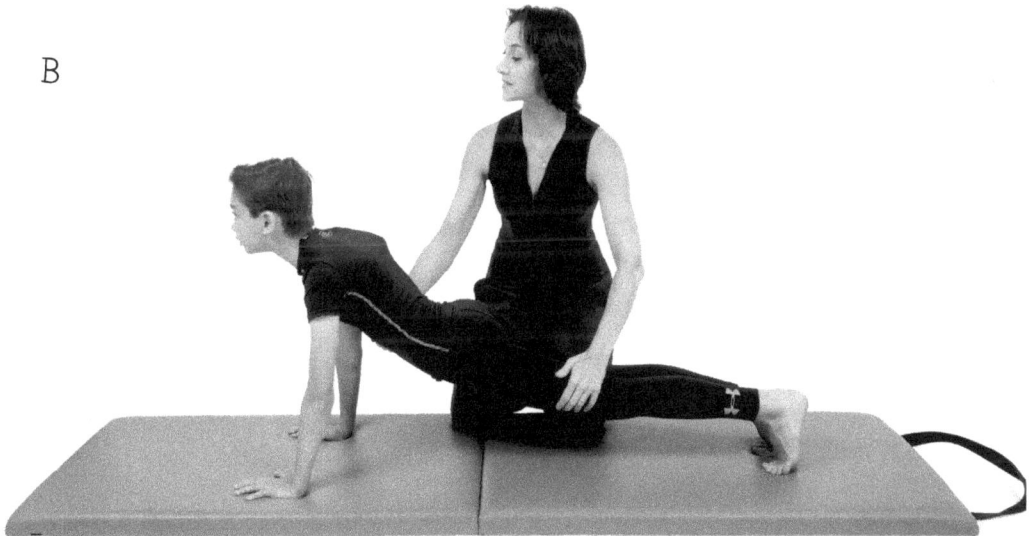

Elephant

An elephant's trunk is a combination of his nose and upper lip. Elephants use their trunks to smell, dig, grasp, touch, gather food, throw dust over their bodies, greet friends, threaten enemies, and siphon water. Elephants suck water part way up their trunks then squirt the water like a hose into their mouths to swallow. Elephants can drink up to fifty gallons of water a day.

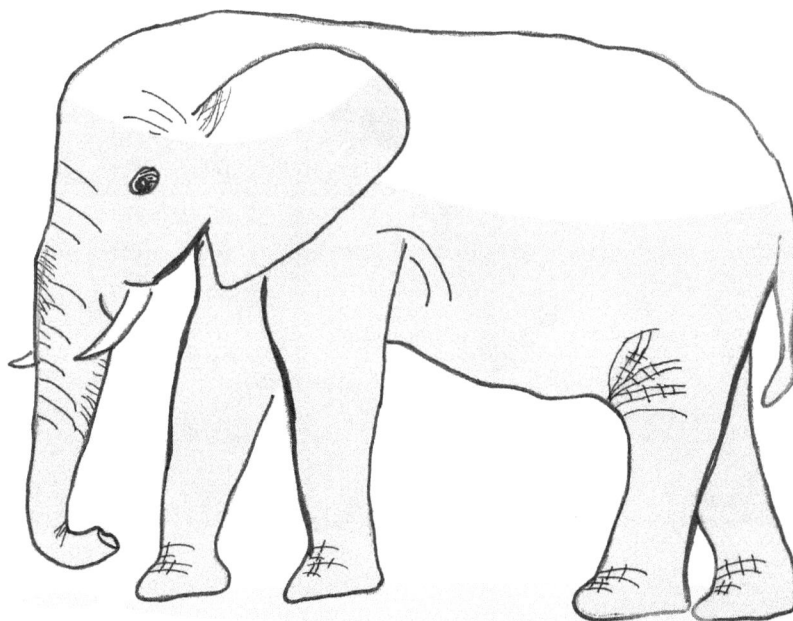

Elephant Walk

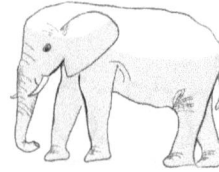

Starting Out

- Stand with your feet parallel and apart.

- Place your hands on the floor in front of your feet.

- *To keep tension out of your neck, let your head hang like the trunk of an elephant gathering food off the ground.*

- Although the goal is to have the palms flat on the floor with the knees straight, you may start out with the fingertips on the floor and/or the legs slightly bent. **Photo A**

- Without moving your arms, shuffle your feet forward and backward while keeping your legs stretched as much as possible.

- Perform 3 times.

A

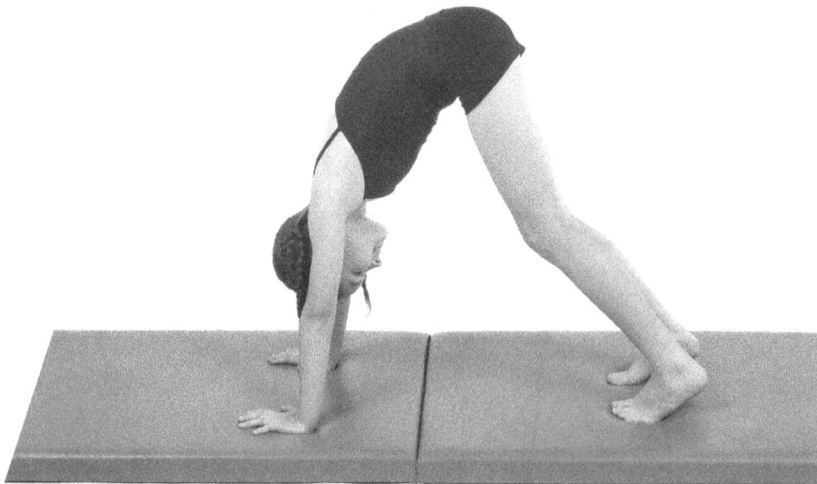

Deeper Practice

- As your strength and flexibility improve, you can walk on all fours.

- As your right hand steps forward, your right leg steps forward. **Photo B**

- As your left hand steps forward, your left leg steps forward.

- Take 6-8 steps, then roll up to standing.

B

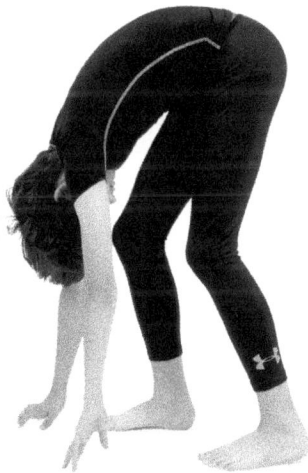

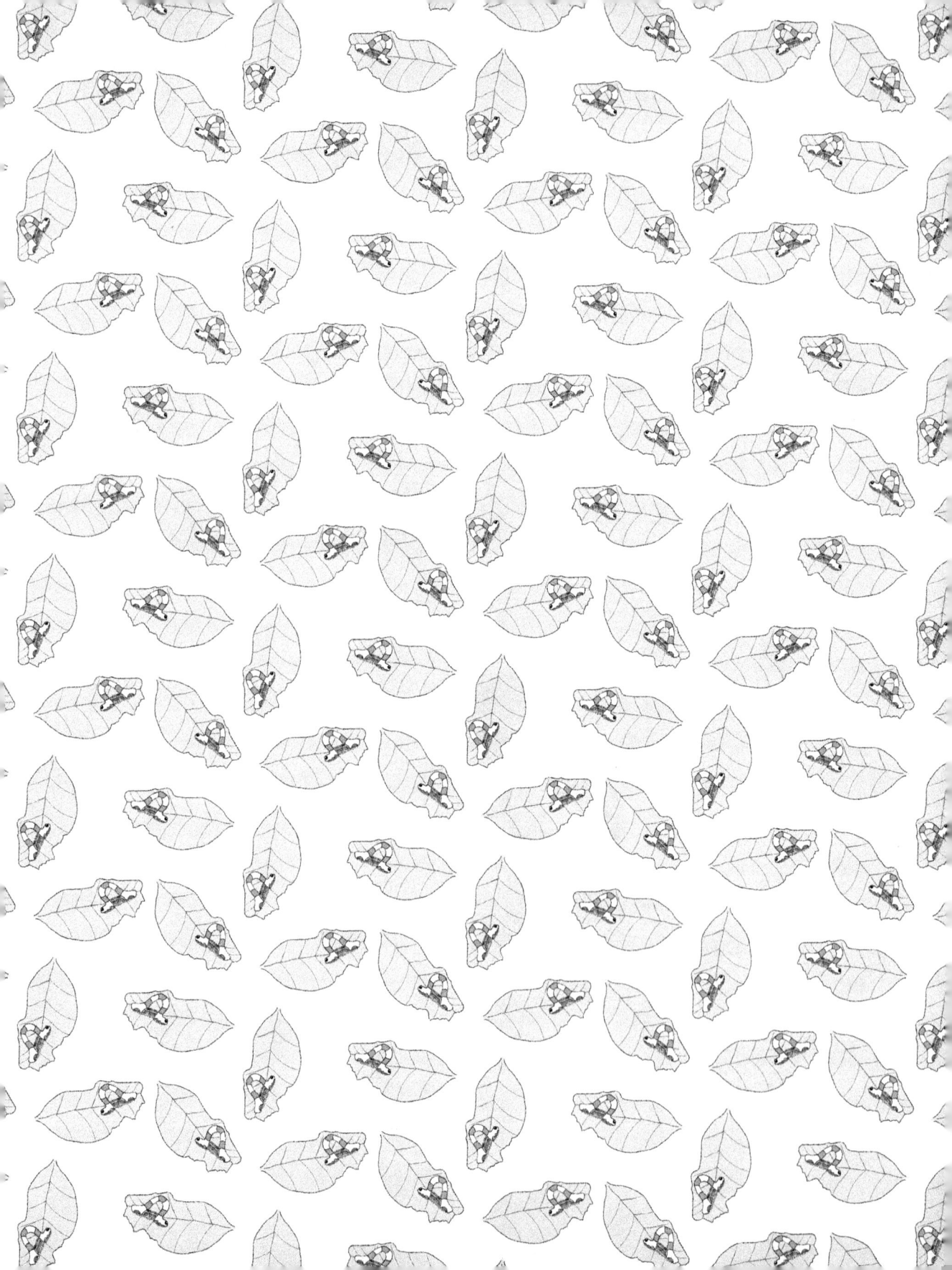

Inchworm

An inchworm is a kind of caterpillar that alternates between stretching its body out long and arching its body as it shifts its weight from one end to the other. Some inchworms can spin silk like a spider when a predator is near. They use the strand of silk to drop quickly from the leaves they are feeding on, and when the danger has passed, they climb back up the silk thread and continue eating. Inchworms eventually turn into moths.

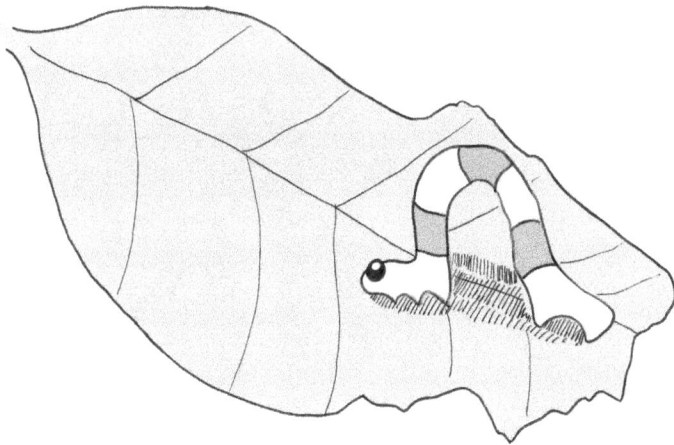

Inchworm Walk

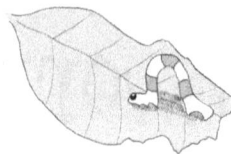

Starting Out

- From the standing position, reach for your toes and walk your hands forward on the floor in four steps, going into a plank shape with your heels together. **Photo A**

- From the plank shape, separate your heels and walk four steps forward on the balls of your feet with stretched legs as your head hangs and your waist lifts. **Photo B**

- Do your best to keep your limbs stretched throughout the movement. *As you shift your weight from your hands to your feet, imagine that you are an inchworm, with legs at both ends of your body and none in the middle.*

- Repeat the sequence 2-3 more times.

Deeper Practice

- For an added challenge, pause in the plank shape and perform one to three push-ups before walking your feet in.

A

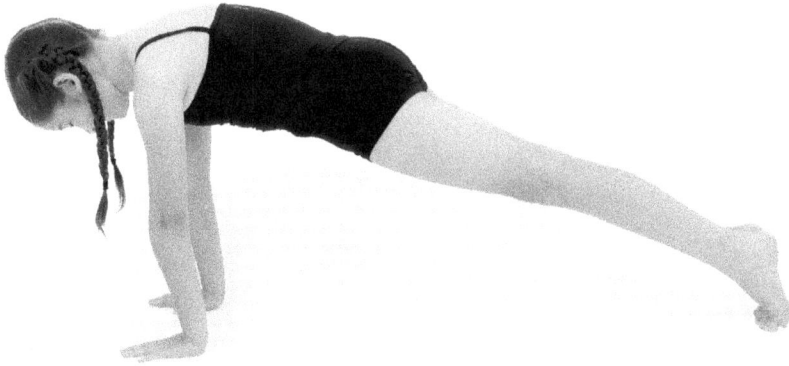

B

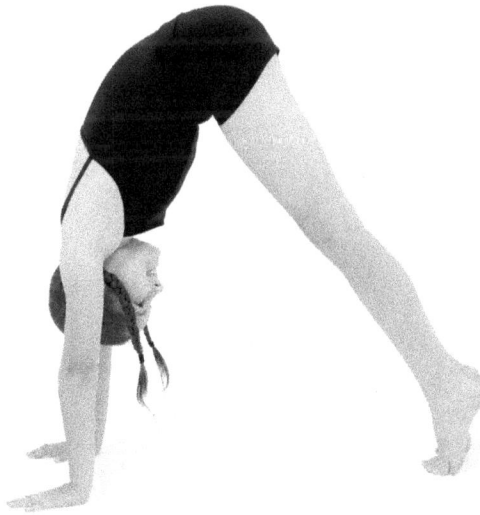

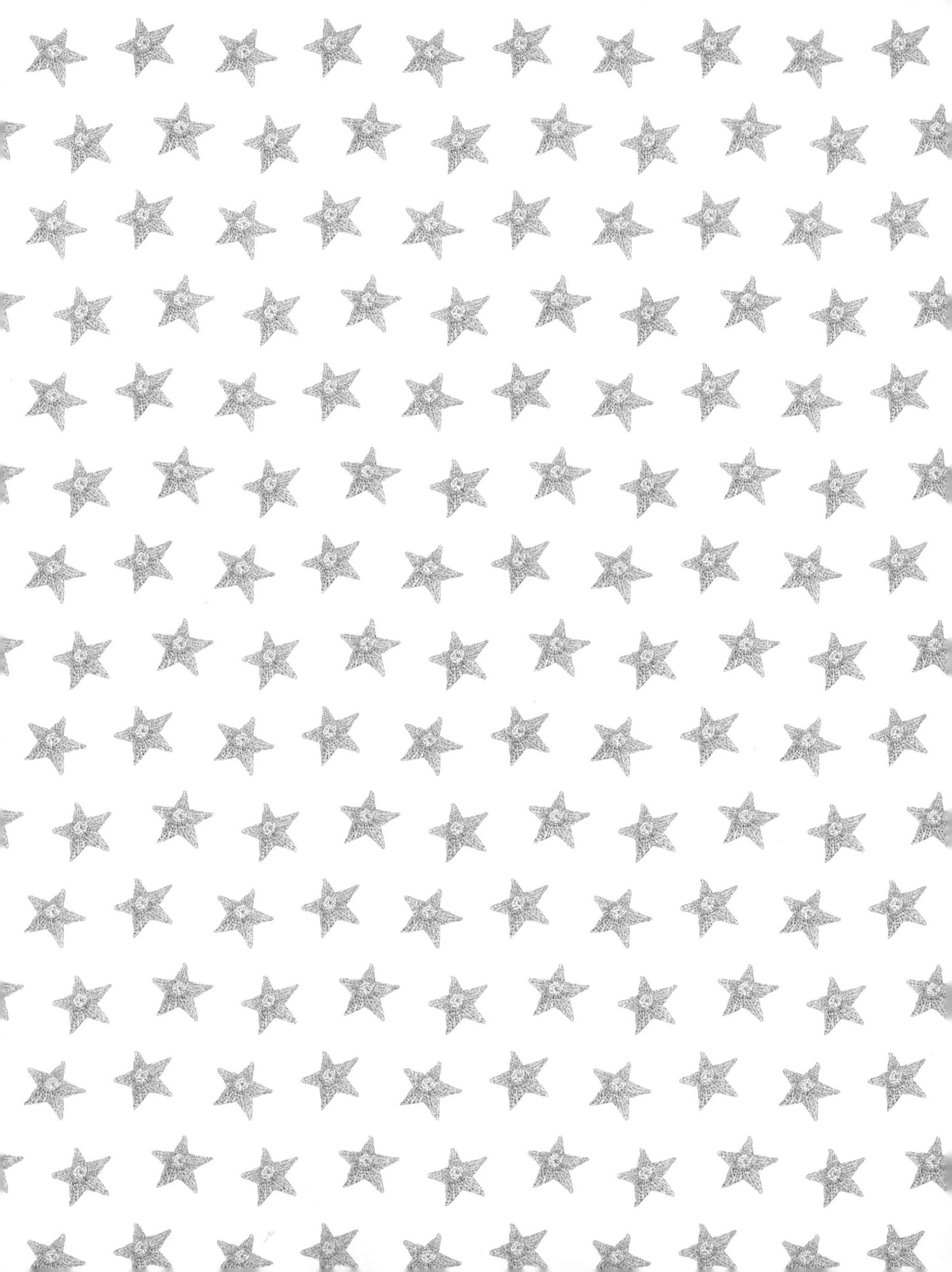

Starfish

Mollusk fishermen used to cut starfish into pieces to kill them because the starfish would get caught in their nets and eat all their mollusks. After cutting the starfish into pieces, the fishermen would toss the pieces into the water. However, instead of killing the starfish, they were creating more of them because each starfish piece became a whole starfish. The fishermen did not realize that starfish can regenerate.

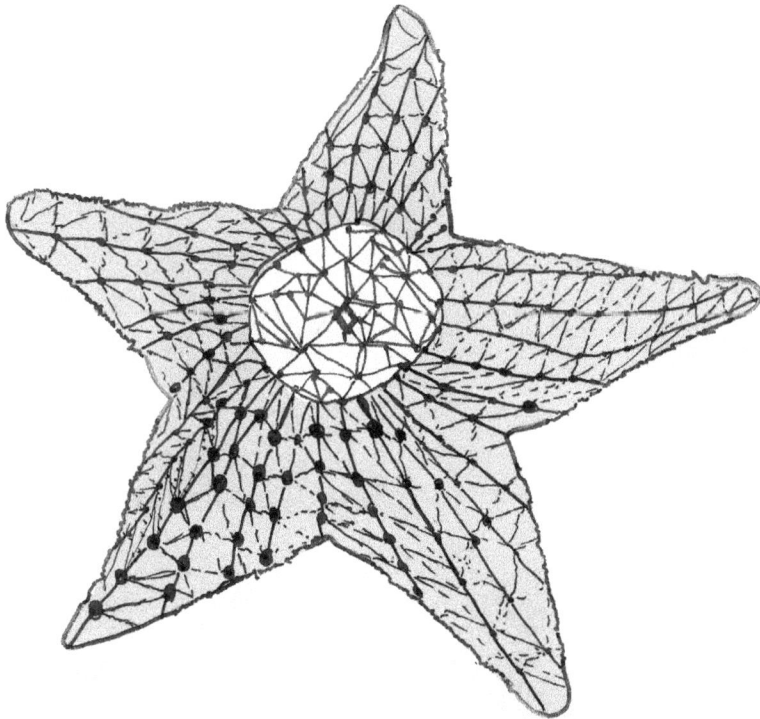

Five-Pointed Starfish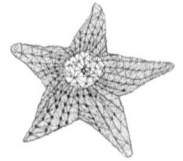

Starting Out

- Begin in a plank position, creating a firm line from the crown of your head to your heels. **Photo A**

- Transition into a side plank shape by moving your right hand in toward your midline and rotating your body to your left.

- As you rotate your body to your left, roll to the outer border of your right foot and bring your left arm long by your side. **Photo B**

- Raise your left arm toward the ceiling and lift your supporting side higher. **Photo C**

- After holding the side plank shape for up to three seconds, return to the plank shape with both hands and feet on the floor.

- Repeat on the other side.

A

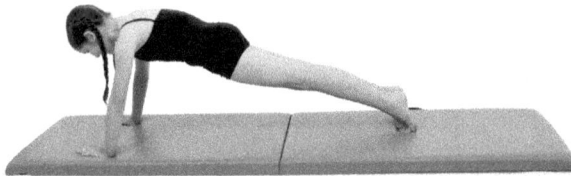

B

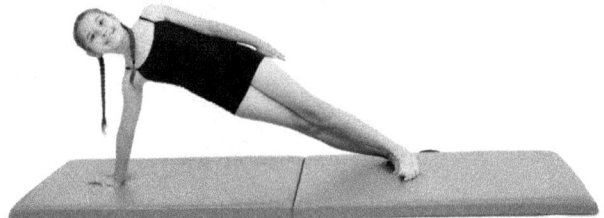

C

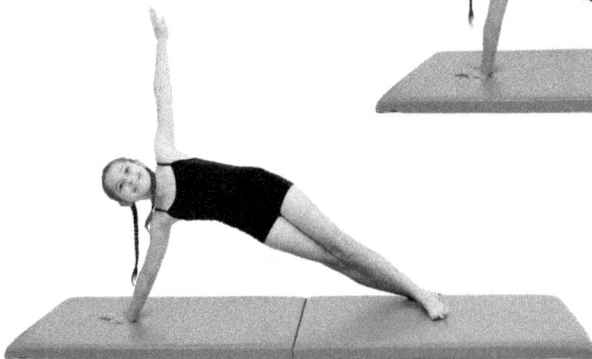

Deeper Practice

- Begin in a plank position, creating a firm line from the crown of your head to your heels. **Photo A**

- Transition into a side plank shape by moving your right hand in toward your midline and rotating your body to your left.

- As you rotate your body to your left, roll to the outer border of your right foot and bring your left arm long by your side. **Photo D**

- Lift the top arm and the top leg toward the ceiling while in the side plank shape. **Photo E**

- *As you reach through the crown of your head and your four limbs, pretend that you are a starfish with five limbs reaching in different directions.*

- Remember to transition through the plank shape between sides.

- Repeat on the other side.

D

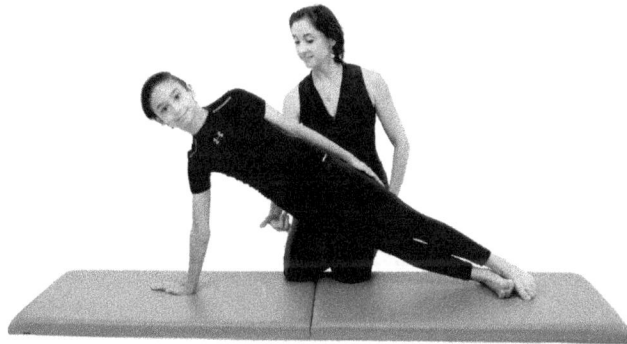

E

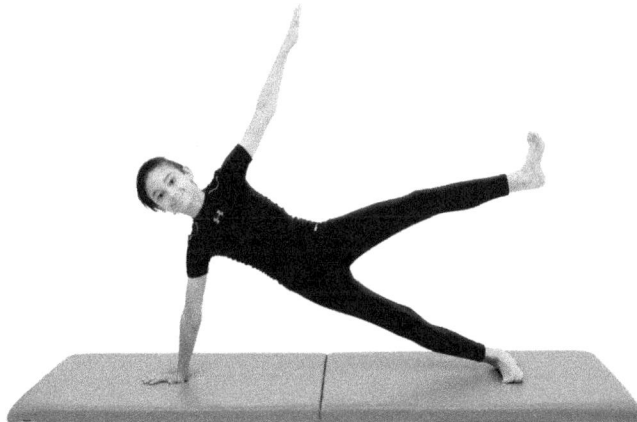

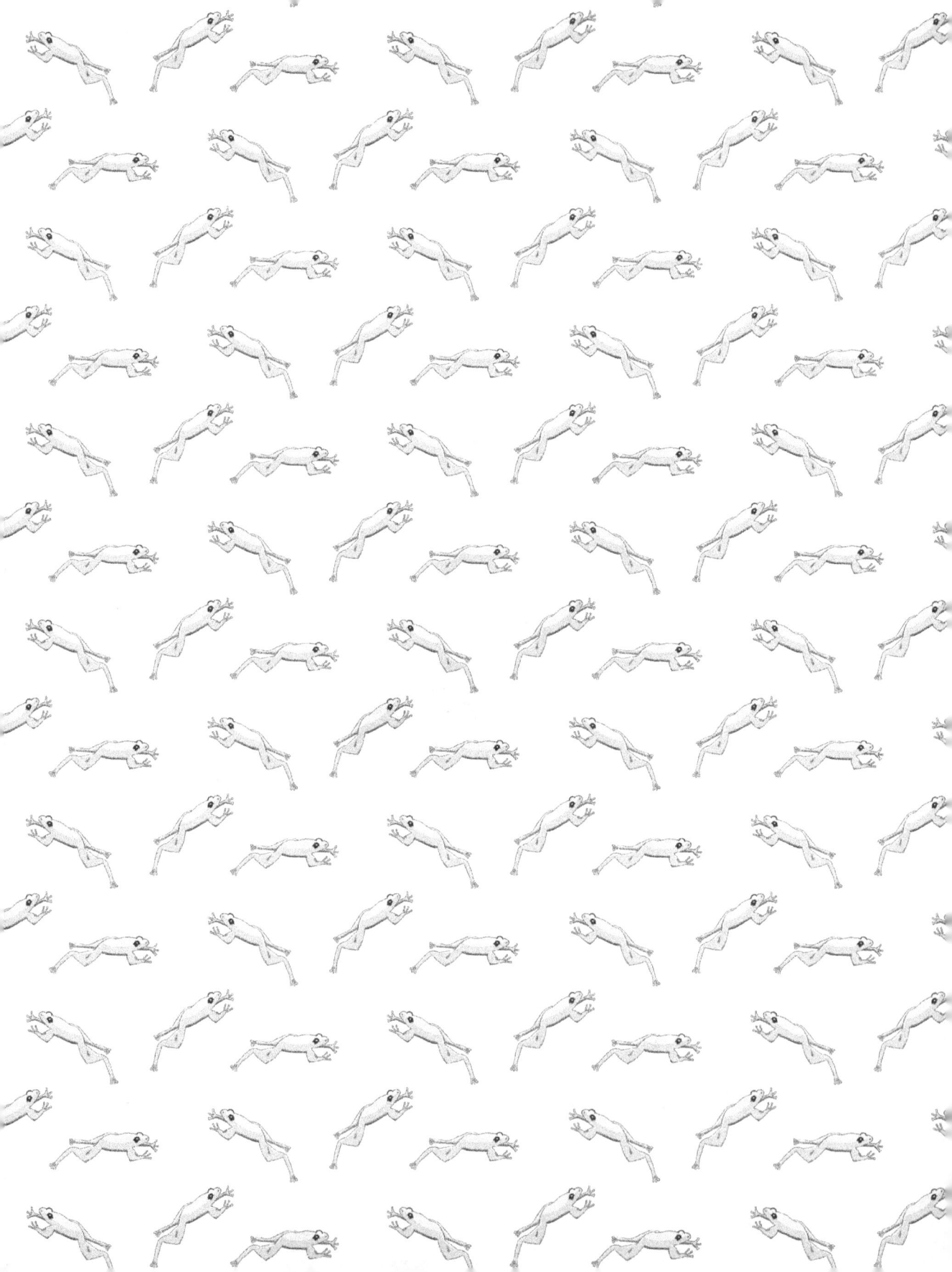

Frog

Different species of frogs have different ways of caring for their fertilized eggs and tadpoles. A female marsupial frog keeps her eggs in a pouch like a kangaroo. When the eggs hatch into tadpoles, the female opens her pouch with her toes and drops them in the water. A male Darwin frog swallows his tadpoles and keeps them in his vocal sac for several months as they grow. When they have transformed, he coughs up tiny, live frogs.

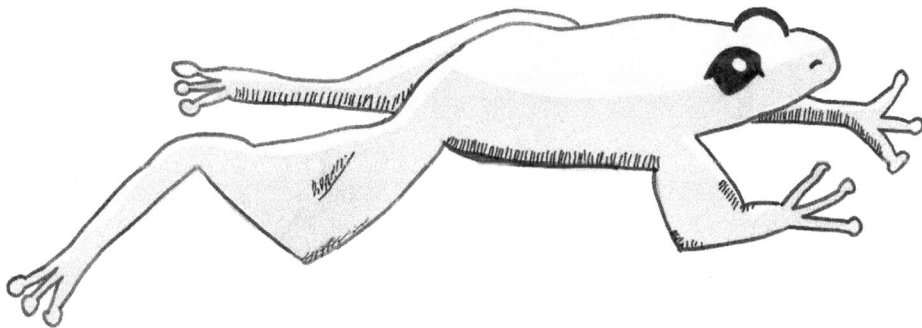

Frog Legs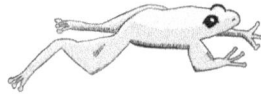

Starting Out

- Stand with your feet in a V shape, heels together, toes apart.

- Open your arms out to the side, and stack your hands behind your head. **Photo A**

- Keep the middle of each knee in line with the toes of each foot as you do a deep knee bend, letting your heels lift as your knee bend gets deeper. Pause three times on the way down and three times on the way up. **Photo B**

- Once standing with the heels on the floor, open your arms in a V-shape overhead before lowering your arms down by your sides.

- *As you bend and stretch your legs, imagine that you are a long-legged frog preparing to jump away from a predator.*

- Perform 1-2 knee bends.

A

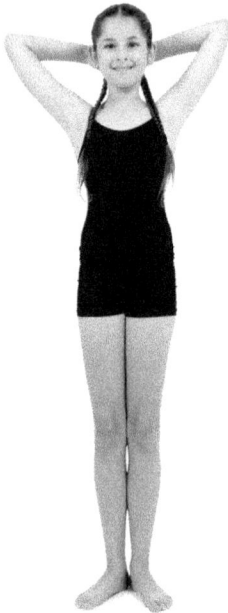

B

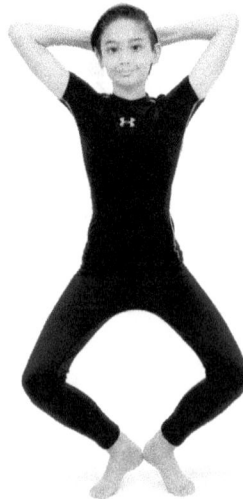

Deeper Practice

- For an added challenge, begin the Frog Legs exercise on the half toe with your heels glued together and toes apart. **Photo C**

- Perform 1-2 knee bends on the half toe, pausing three times on the way down and three times on the way up. **Photo D**

- Staying on the half toe throughout the knee bend can be a challenge, so remember to keep your heels glued together to help find your midline and hold your balance.

C

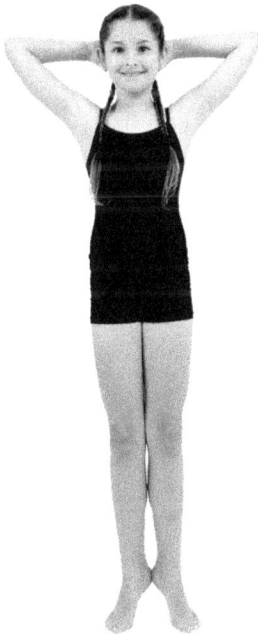

D

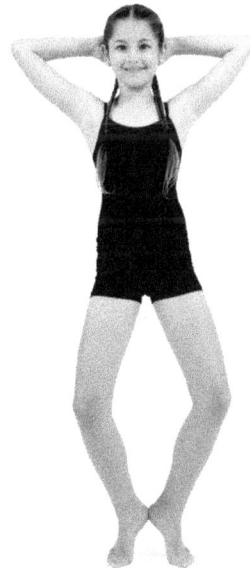

Horse

It only takes one to two hours for a newborn horse to stand up and walk. Baby horses, called foals, are born with their legs almost the same length as those of adults, which makes it extra challenging for them to reach down and eat grass.

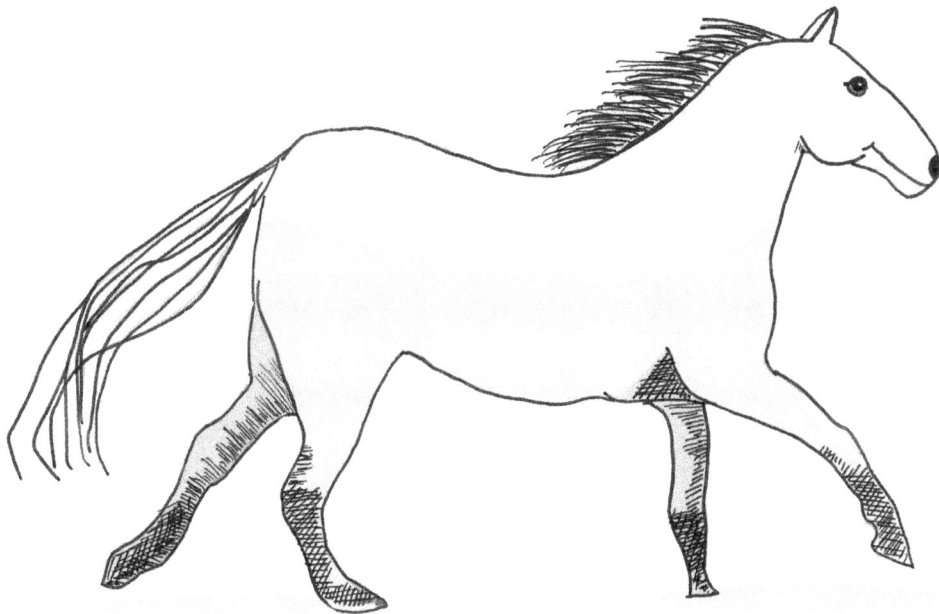

Horse Prancing

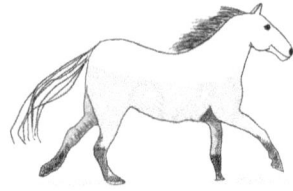

Starting Out

- Stand on the floor with your feet parallel and slightly apart.

- Place your hands on your hips as a reminder to keep your hips even.

- Rise to the half toe with straight legs. **Photo A**

- Lower one heel to the floor with a straight leg, and lift the opposite heel higher as that leg bends. **Photo B**

- *As you alternate lifting each heel, imagine you are a horse prancing. To keep the movement light and bouncy, imagine that your bellybutton is a rubber ball rebounding off the floor.*

- Prance 20 times.

Deeper Practice

- To challenge your balance control, add a small hold after every three prances, when both feet are on the half toe and both legs are straight. **Photo A**

A

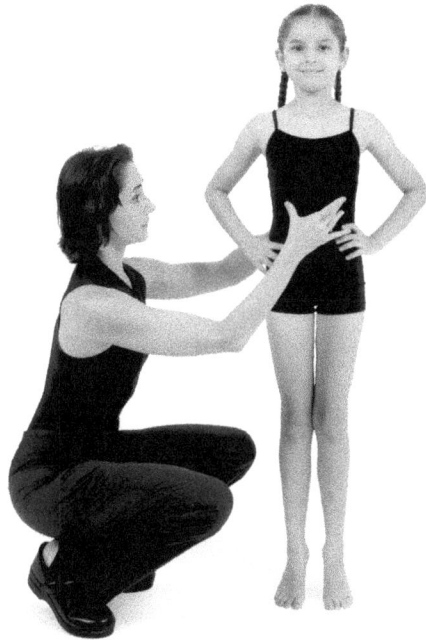

B

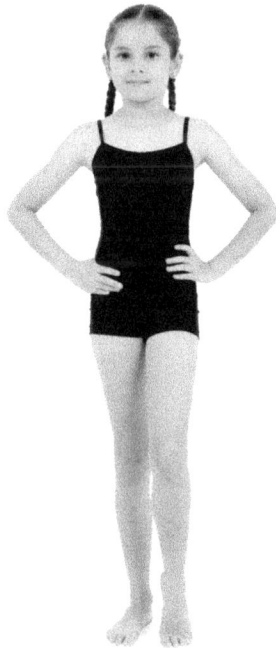

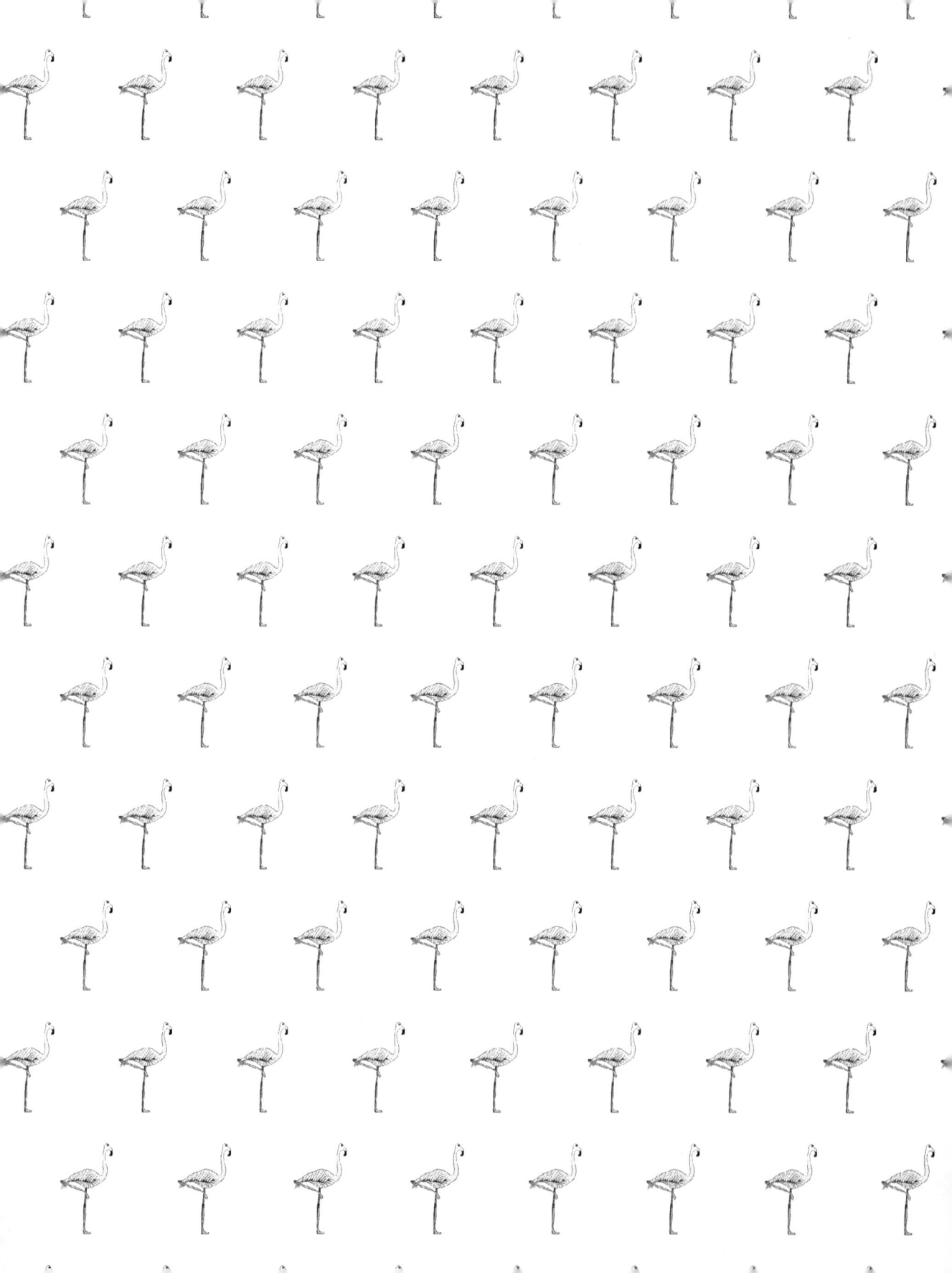

Flamingo

Flamingos often stand on one leg with the other leg tucked under the body. The bend in their leg appears to be their knee joint, but is actually their ankle joint. Their knee is much higher on the leg. Flamingos can balance on one leg for hours and even sleep standing on one leg. A flamingo's ankle joint, the one where you would expect the knee to be, can lock into position when the leg is straight. This locking mechanism may explain why flamingos have such incredible balance on one leg.

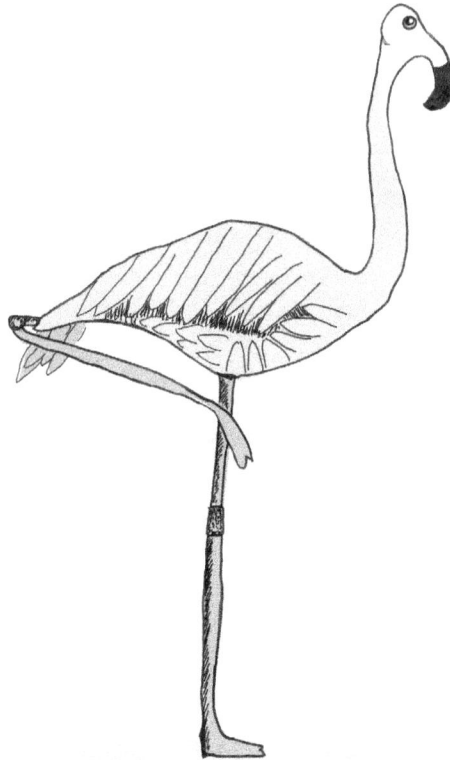

Pink Flamingo

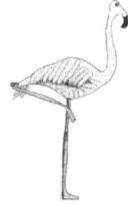

Starting Out

- Stand tall with your forearms stacked and elbows lifted.
- Keep your hips and shoulders even as you alternate lifting one knee at a time. **Photo A**
- Perform up to 20 knee lifts.

Deeper Practice

- For an extra challenge, balance for three seconds on one leg on every third knee lift.
- *Imagine you are a flamingo whose balance is better on one leg than it is on two.*

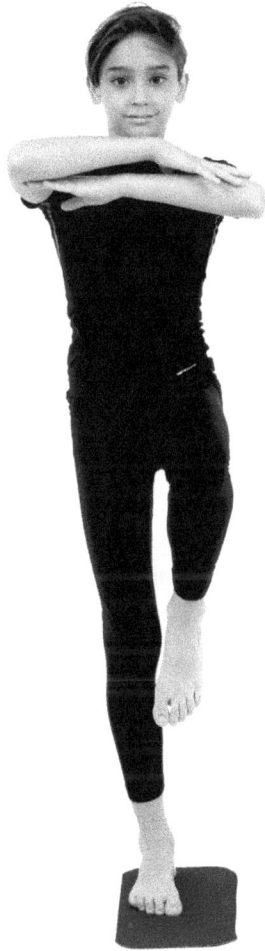

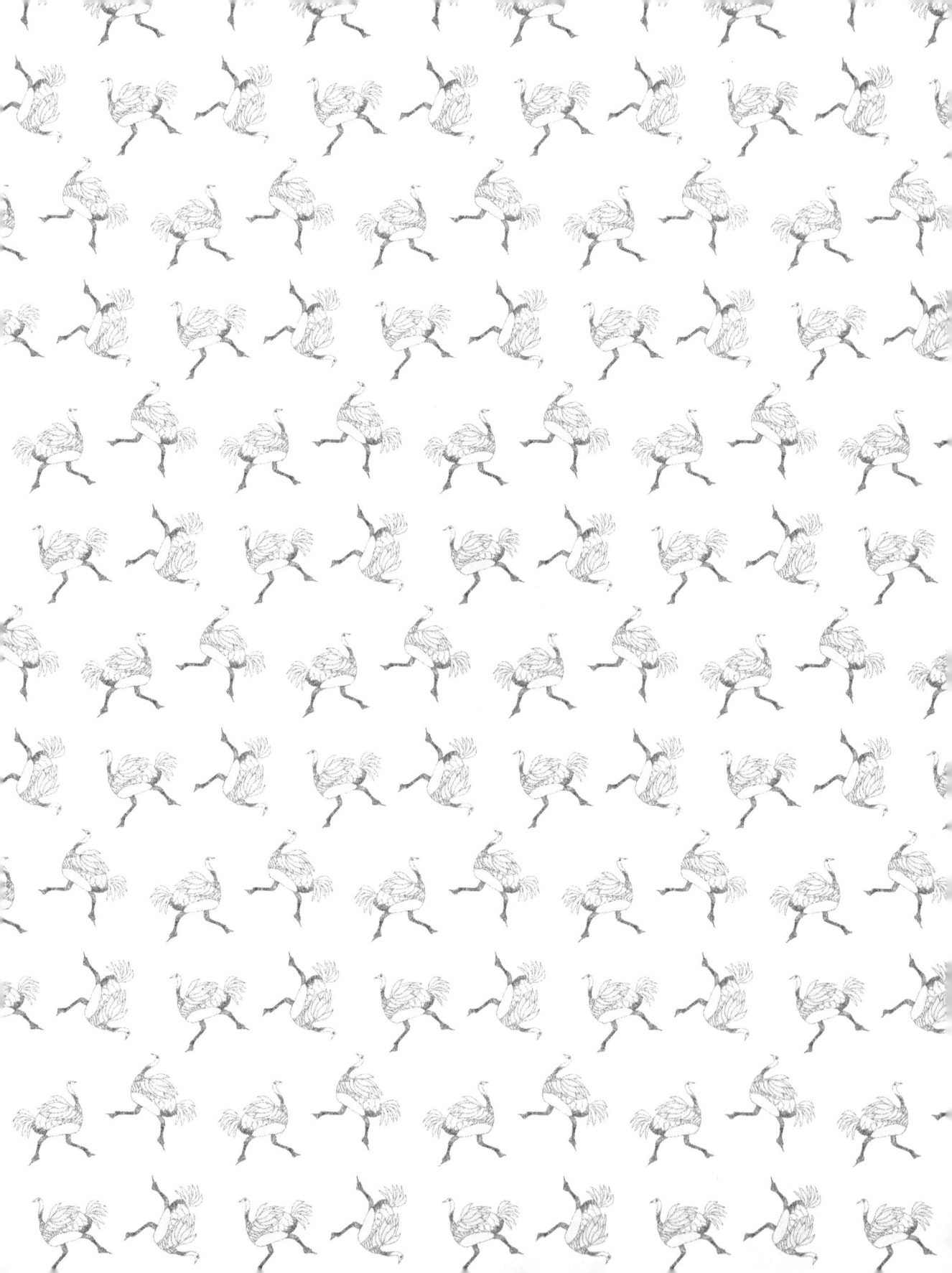

Ostrich

Although the ostrich is a bird, it does not fly. It is the fastest bird on land and the fastest animal on two legs. It can run just over 40 miles an hour. To maintain its balance, the ostrich stretches its short wings out to the side as it runs. In addition to running, an ostrich uses its legs for self-defense. It has enough power in its legs to kill a lion with its kick.

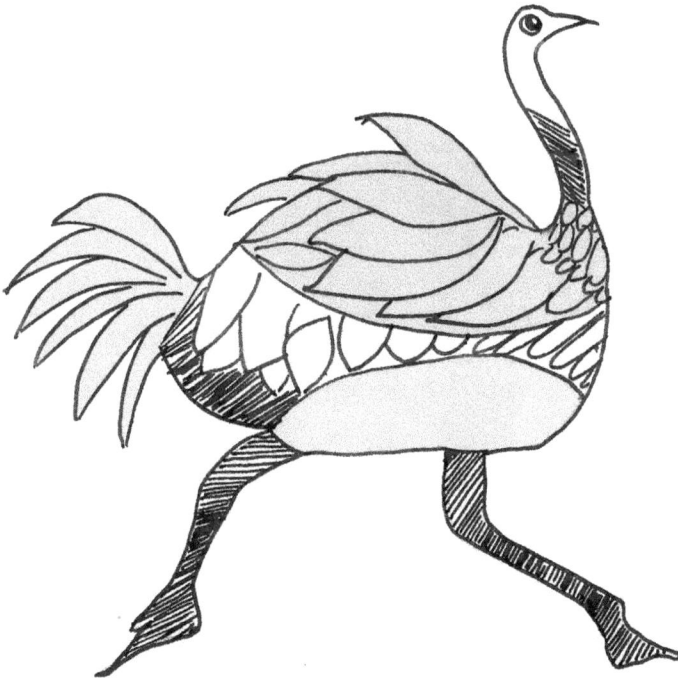

Running Ostrich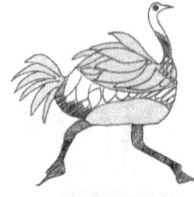

Starting Out

- Stand tall and extend your arms out to the side.
- Lift the heel of one foot toward your seat, and bend your supporting leg to begin jogging in place.
- Try to kick your heels to your seat. **Photo A**
- Perform 1-3 sets of eight heel kicks to the seat.

A

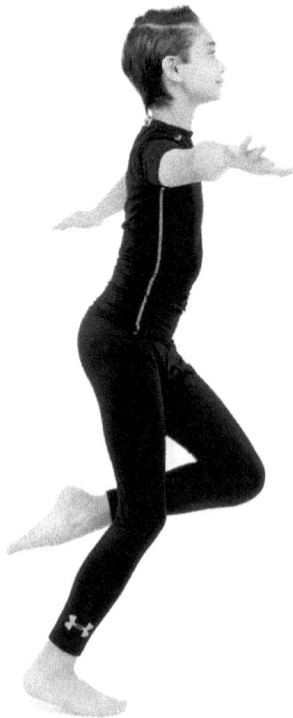

Deeper Practice

- If space allows, you can run the perimeter of the room while trying to kick your heels into your seat.

- *As you run with outstretched arms, imagine you are an ostrich with powerful legs.* **Photo B**

- The number of laps depends on the size of your room.

B

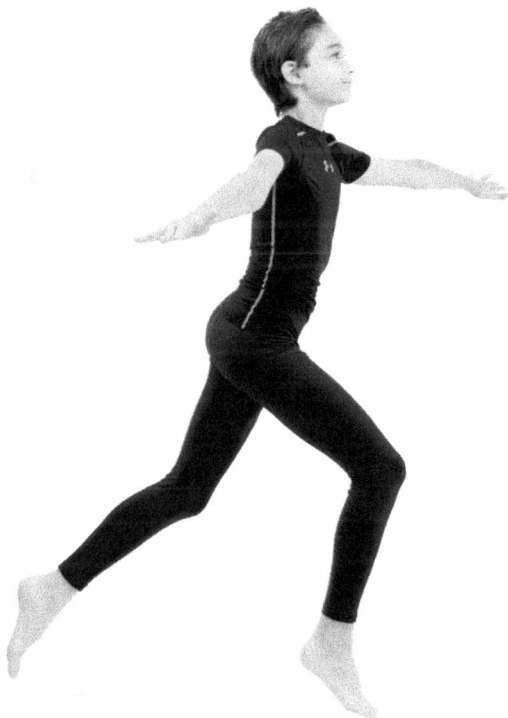

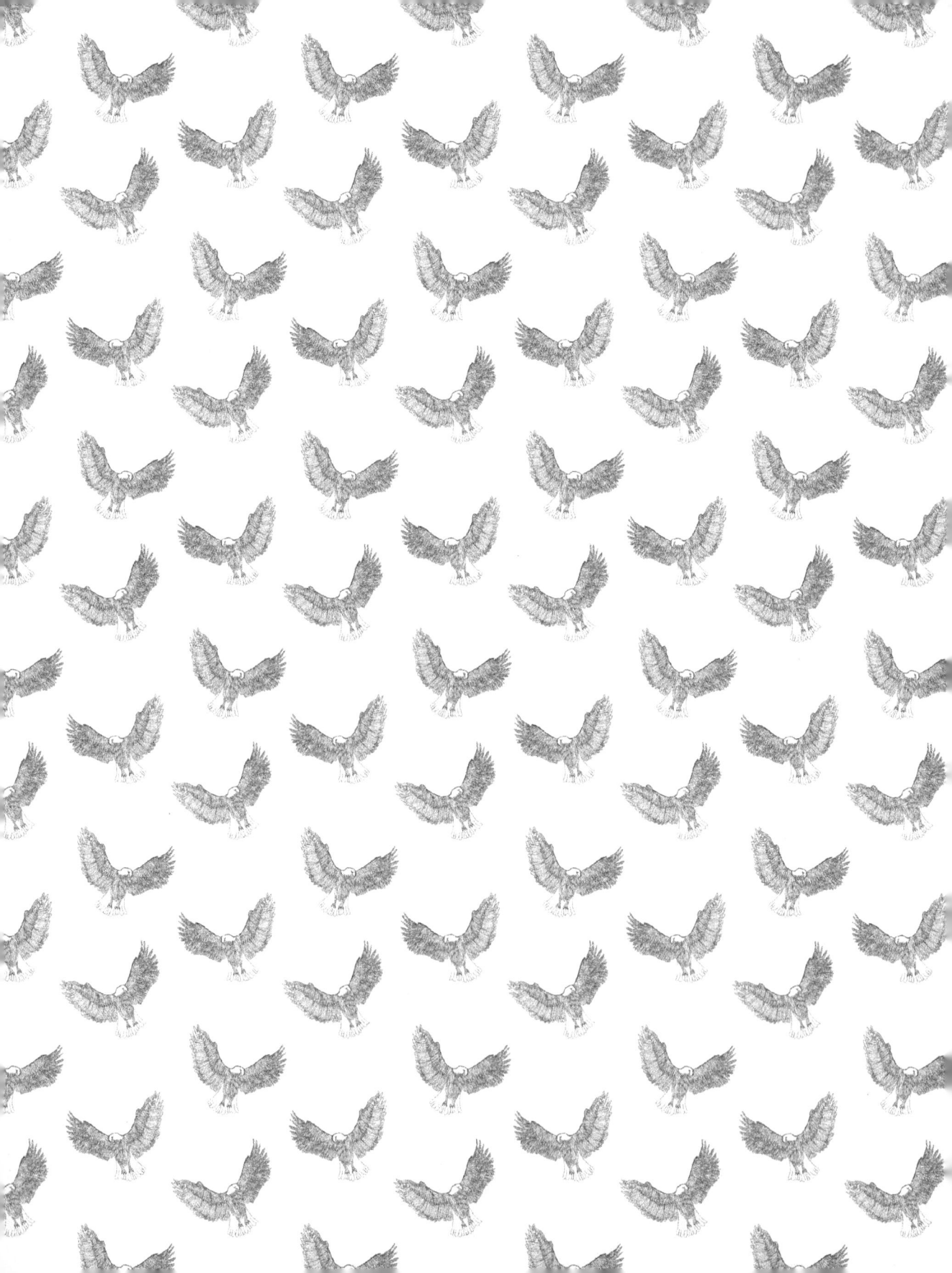

Eagle

Unlike hawks and vultures that soar with their wings in a slight V-shape, eagles soar with their wings straight out. Sometimes bald eagles grab each other's feet (talons) while flying and spin toward the ground with their talons locked together. It is not known whether they are fighting or playing, but if they do not separate before hitting the ground, they can be injured.

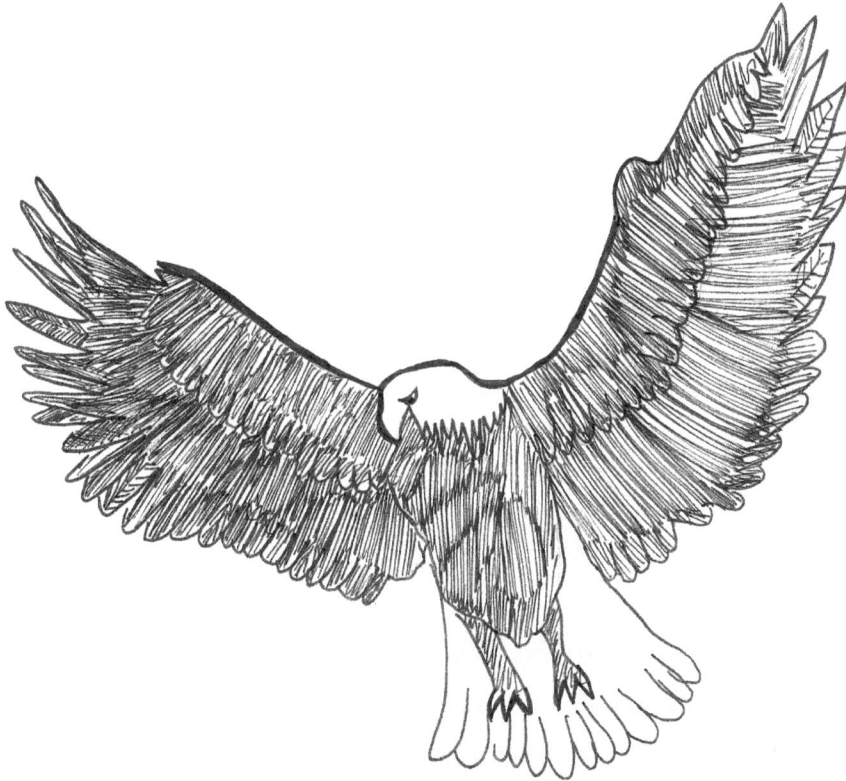

Proud Eagle

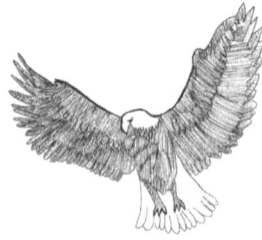

Starting Out

- Stand tall with your bellybutton pulled in and up.

- Feet can be together in "eagle stance" with the heels together and the toes apart, in a V shape.

- Take a deep breath and lift your arms in front of you in a closed hug position.

- Continue to breathe in and lift your arms so that they frame your face. **Photo A**

- Breathe out as your arms open to the side, palms facing the floor. **Photo B**

- *Imagine that you are an eagle soaring through the sky as you spread your wings.*

- Perform 3 times.

A

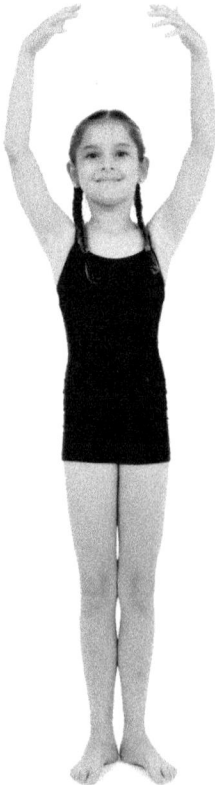

B

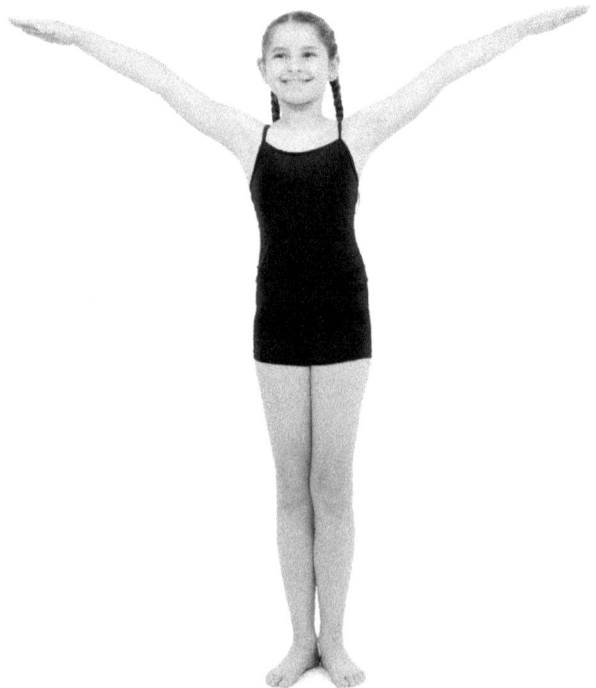

Deeper Practice

- Begin standing tall in "eagle" stance with your arms down by your sides.
- Fold in half and reach for your toes. **Photo C**
- Extend your arms forward as you lift your torso parallel to the floor. **Photo D**
- Stand upright as your arms frame your face. **Photo E**
- As your arms open to the side, palms facing upward, lift your chest toward the ceiling and go into a small backbend in your upper back, finishing with your arms down by your sides. **Photo F**
- Perform 2-3 large arm circles.

C

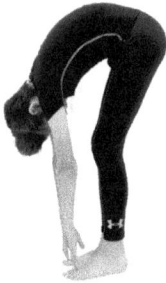

D

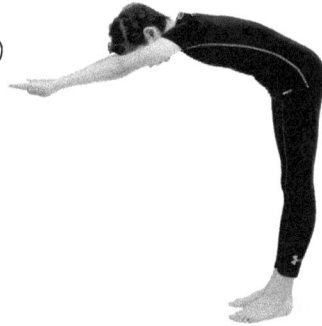

E

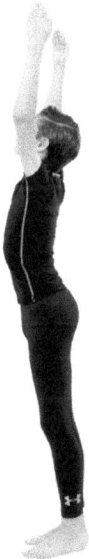

F

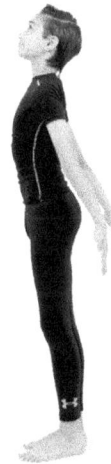

Congratulations on completing the Pilates Animals Workout®!

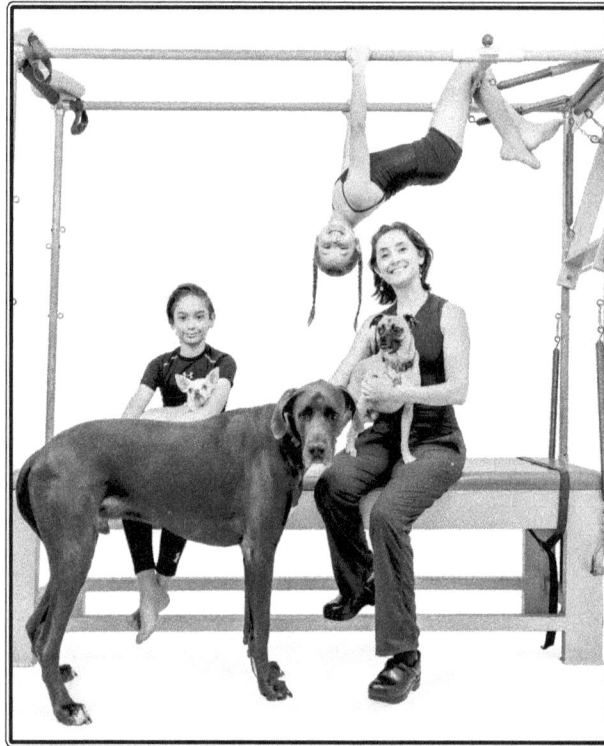

A BIG thank you to:

My creative daughter, whose animal drawings inspired me
to write this book,

My talented son, who encouraged me to teach his basketball
team weekly conditioning classes and whose invaluable advice
helped me refine the Pilates Animals Workout®,

My photographer Max Kelly,
for his patience during our long photo shoots and his creative
book cover design,

My graphic designer Yael Rotstein Campbell,
for her expertise in the design and layout of this book's interior,

And Judith Rock,
for her invaluable editing.

I also wish to thank:

My husband and my mother for their endless love and support,

My mentors Fernando Bujones and Romana Kryzanowska,

My teachers and students,

All my children's teachers, especially Zara Baroyan,
Ruth Hershman, Alan Evans, Tommy Brown, Jamil Ghattas,
and Julie Burch,

And to all those who encouraged me not to give up on my belief
that there is value in teaching children Pilates.

Christina Maria Gadar

Author and creator of the Pilates Animals Workout®

I grew up in a household full of pets. At one point, we had a total of twenty cats in addition to dogs, rabbits, chinchillas, guinea pigs, hamsters, gerbils, mice, gecko lizards, a rescued lab rat named Cleopatra, and a pot-bellied pig that ended up weighing nearly 300 pounds! In addition to our pets, we always had some form of wildlife undergoing rehabilitation in one of our bathrooms. I'll never forget the day I found a wild goose in our bathtub! Growing up with so many animals gave me an appreciation for their sincerity, intelligence, and their intuitiveness about their bodies. I created the Pilates Animals Workout®, or P.A.W. for short, because I wanted to create a Pilates workout for children that would leave them feeling as fit as animals.

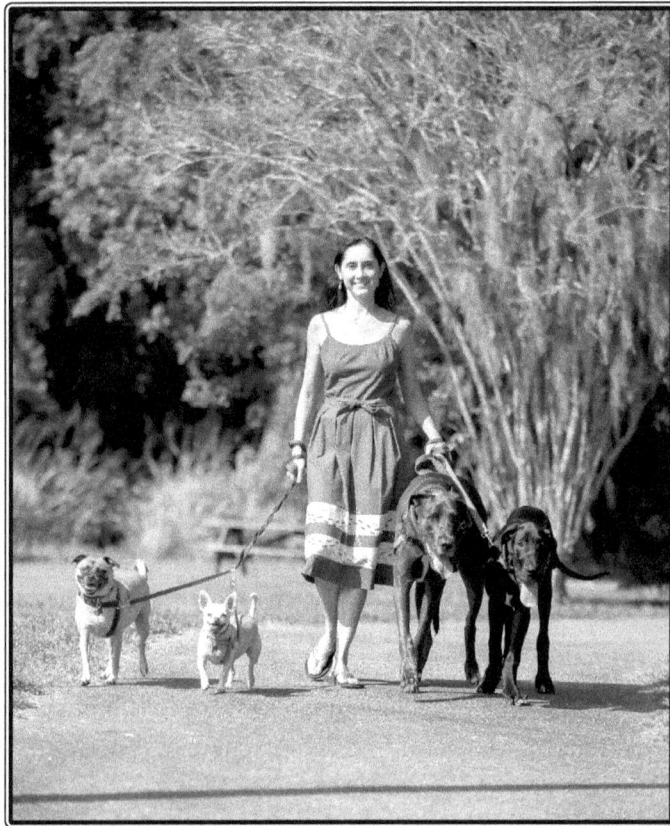

Taís Haydée Gadar
Illustrator and model

I love my pets because they give me love and bring me joy. No matter how I'm feeling, they always manage to put a smile on my face. It's not always easy having a house full of pets. Especially when my two Great Danes take up all the space on the sofa, or when my Chihuahua tries to steal my food, but the more I have animals in my life, the more I cherish them.

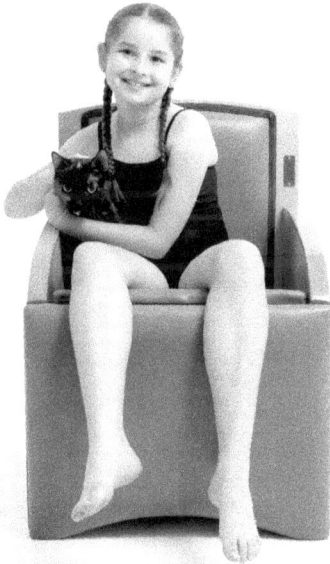

Marcelo Gadar
Model

I love my pets because they are genuine, playful, and kind. But what some people don't know is that they are very musical too. My Chihuahua and Pug always sing when my sister plays the trumpet and my Great Dane puppy always steps on the piano bench and tries to touch the keys during my piano lessons. It is hard work having pets, but it's okay because animals are a huge part of my life.

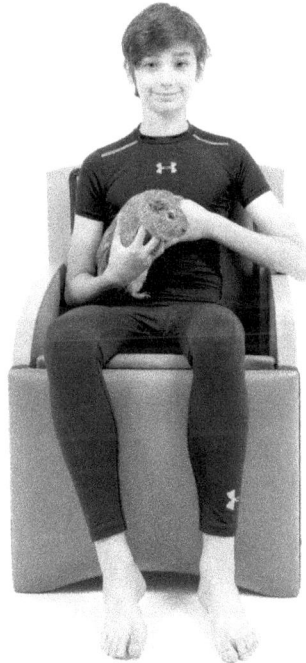

> *"All creatures swell to magnificence when seen through the lens of a child's eye."*

Edward O. Wilson
Biologist and Pulitzer prize winning author

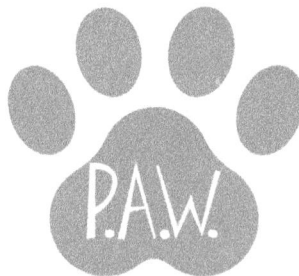

P.A.W.

Pilates Animals Workout®

References

Archival Footage of Joseph Pilates. Historical film footage compiled and edited by Power Pilates, 2005.

Baldwin, Mary Burt. "Gym Owner Has Youthful Glow at 83." *New York Times,* 12 April 1963, p. 43.

Brown, Beth. "How to Stay Fit Lying Down." *Pageant,* Nov. 1963, pp. 128-133.

Joseph H. Pilates: Demonstrating the Principles of his Method with Clara, Students and Friends. Archival film footage compiled and edited by Mary Bowen from Joe Pilates' private film collection, 1932-1945.

Pilates, Joseph H. *Return to Life Through Contrology.* 1945. The Christopher Publishing House, 1960.

Trier, Carola S. *Exercise: What It Is, What It Does.* Greenwillow Books, 1982.

Wernick, Robert. "To Keep in Shape: Act Like an Animal." *Sports Illustrated*, east coast edition, 12 Feb. 1962, pp. E5-E8.

---. "To Keep in Shape: Act Like an Animal." *Sports Illustrated*, unedited edition, 12 Feb. 1962, www.pilates.org.au/joseph-pilates-act-like-an-animal/. Accessed 14 April 2015

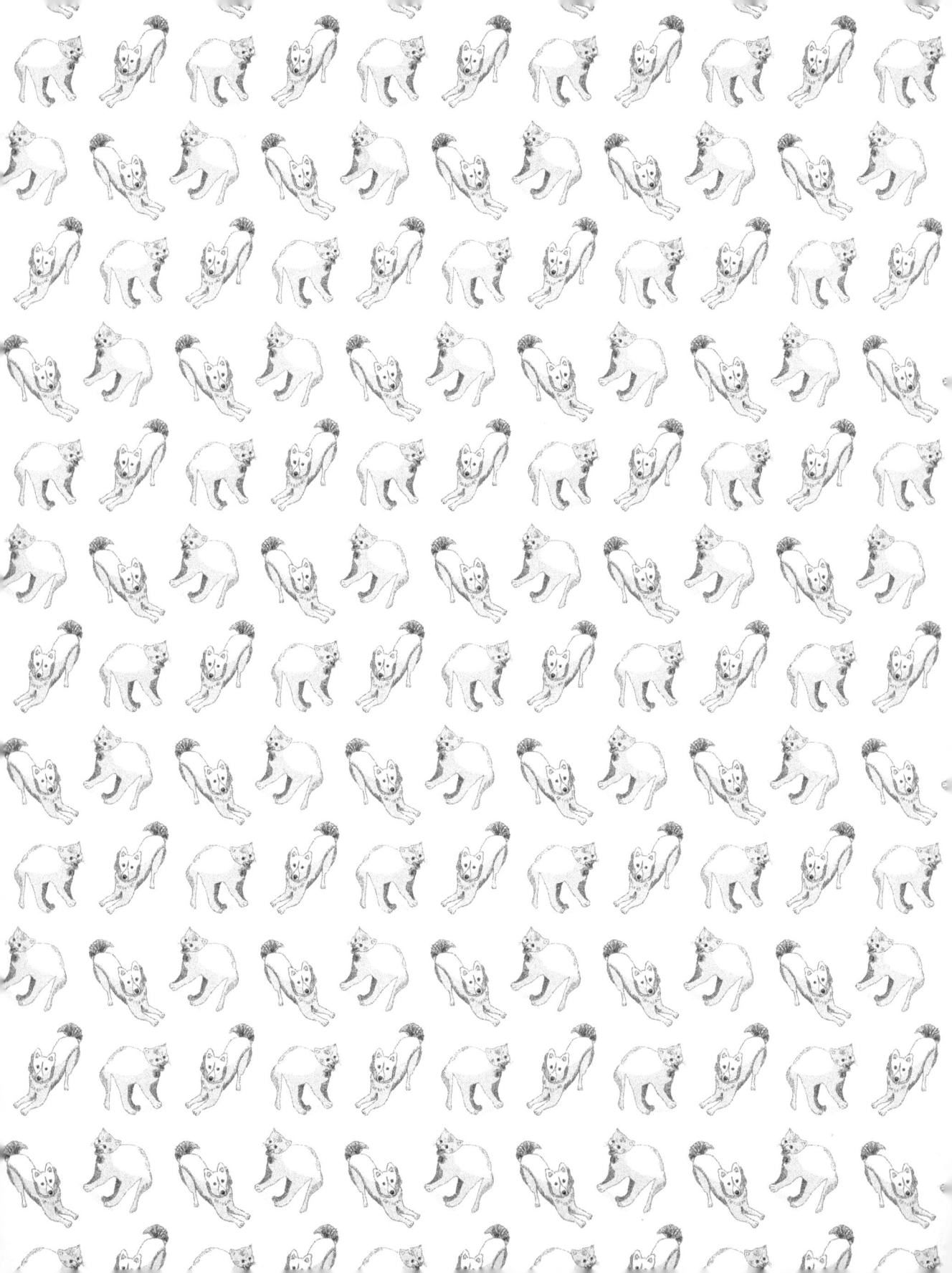

www.ingramcontent.com/pod-product-compliance
Lightning Source LLC
Chambersburg PA
CBHW080242270326
41926CB00020B/4342